# Stress Is A Choice

## Taking Responsibility For Our Natural Life.

**Brian  A. Ling**

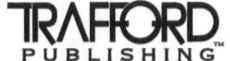

TRAFFORD
PUBLISHING™

Front Cover Photograph by Brian Ling.

Note for Librarians: A cataloguing record for this book is available from Library and Archives Canada at www.collectionscanada.ca/amicus/index-e.html
ISBN 1-4120-9370-8

*Trafford's print shop runs on "green energy" from solar, wind and other environmentally-friendly power sources.*

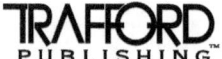
**PUBLISHING™**
*Offices in Canada, USA, Ireland and UK*

**Book sales for North America and international:**
Trafford Publishing, 6E–2333 Government St.,
Victoria, BC V8T 4P4 CANADA
phone 250 383 6864 (toll-free 1 888 232 4444)
fax 250 383 6804; email to orders@trafford.com
**Book sales in Europe:**
Trafford Publishing (UK) Limited, 9 Park End Street, 2nd Floor
Oxford, UK OX1 1HH UNITED KINGDOM
phone +44 (0)1865 722 113 (local rate 0845 230 9601)
facsimile +44 (0)1865 722 868; info.uk@trafford.com
**Order online at:**
trafford.com/06-1124

10 9 8 7 6 5 4 3 2

# Contents

# *Introduction*

We are living busier and more complicated lives than ever. We are caught in a society that is lunging forward at greater speeds and dragging each of us with it. More people are feeling isolated and see their lives out of control with more expectations placed upon them. There is a sense of helplessness drifting through the hearts of many. Each of us is affected by others. We don't know what to do. This book is for those people.

Some say this is the age of technology, which is supposed to give us more time and energy for ourselves. For many it drains us to an even further extent. As individuals we must step in and intervene. We need to advocate for ourselves and take control of our lives. As each individual regains their life, we all do.

The book offers no simple answers. It is about asking the reader to take complete responsibility for their life. It is about looking at our lives in ways we may never have before. It is about seriously looking at our addiction to the culture we live in. We are asked to look at the question what is it to be a human being. It is about commitment and hard work. It is about being a trailblazer and taking your own journey. It is about loving life.

This book is a powerful tool that when merged with earnest vigour will bring about remarkable results in successfully managing stress.

Brian

# Chapter 1
# *Daily Living*

The days, weeks, months and years seem to come and go at a faster pace. We often tell ourselves we are accomplishing things, getting them done. There is more to be done so we continue at this pace, eventually increasing the pace to keep up with the new demands. Meals are hurried, eliminated, or simply bought for convenience. Children are rushed to the baby sitter followed by a dash to the office. Politics, professional policy and financial profit orchestrate how we survive the day. What's left of the day is spent trying to fit in a myriad of activities such as going to the gym, attending a meeting, creating family time, and religious practices.

The routine appears to be repeated day after day. During brief interludes thoughts or feelings something is not quite right flash by. Not sure what to make of them and convincing ourselves we don't have time, we dismiss them. After all, we are living the appropriate life because most others are doing the same. The moments of unease, questioning and wonder continue to appear, often when least expected. They persist with an ebb and flow. But we brush them aside. The episodes of momentary awareness of pure joy and happiness we occasionally experienced in the past are becoming fewer.

Yes, this moment-to-moment life we live is for our benefit, our family's, and we are helping the world. Or so we tell ourselves. We are masters at convincing ourselves of almost anything. We have challenging moments through events such as illness, divorce, death and unemployment. When we survive them, we return to our regular routine with even greater speed, desperately trying to escape from the past harrowing experience. We are now even more grateful for the questionable life we have been living for years. Deep within ourselves we are even more afraid. The cycle of daily living we have created continues.

We slowly and methodically have more difficulty verbalizing or feeling what it is we are uncomfortable with. We continue to see people, events and situations differently as time goes on. We treat our closest family members with contempt, anger and frustration. We make more and more demands on them. We create more separation from members of our nuclear family. Our constellation of extended family commitments becomes continuously strained as we search for time or emotional closeness to justify our very family. This life is about my needs, isn't it?

We are bombarded with increasing amounts of commercial advertising every moment of our lives. Confused and unaware, we justify searching for what we are convinced we need while being led by the illusion of security. This list also includes such things as cars, computers, cell phones, new homes, clothing, jewellery or a new job. The daily routine of I need, I seek and I find continues.

We are also bombarded with increasing amounts of professional advertising. Whatever craft we have chosen to make our living with, the emotional weight is increasing as we are engulfed by more outside control. We think we must endure. We are told it is for the protection/benefit of those around us as well as our protection/benefit. We have less choice in how we choose to behave and practice our craft and spend more time meeting the demands of others. This is our day-to-day life. The thoughts and feelings that something is not quite right persist. They do not seem to fit into any paradigm we recognise. We don't know what to do. The dissonance is growing.

We make the decision to strive for promotion so we can dictate to the ones who are in the position we are currently in. This will finally solve our problems. More time and energy is invested in pleasing those who are able to promote us. We make it. We have a new title on the office door and earn more money. Soon it becomes apparent we have more demands upon us. Pleasing those above us as well as pleasing those below us becomes of primary concern. Even less time is spent with family, interests and community. We seldom notice the continuous moments of life flowing by. We don't seem to feel as important as we did at promotion time.

Our religious or spiritual practices will support us. Through obligation, guilt and conditioning we squeeze in time for our regular practice. Interestingly, we pray for someone else to take responsibility for our actions. There continues to be a sense that something is not right. Or, are we just exhausted and lack simple appreciation for this moment.? Where do we turn? There is no answer, or is there?

The latest diet book is published and it is the definitive answer. The latest philosophy for personal transformation is spread by the media. We turn to them. More time and energy is invested draining precious delight from the responsibilities and activities we enjoy. But these were the final answers!

Maybe we are not working hard enough. Colleagues are spending more hours at work than we are, and are suggesting we are not carrying our responsibility. That must be it! Therefore more time is spent at work. Much of the time we question the validity and ethics of what we do. It is of deep concern to us but we do nothing about it. We are told our job is to produce, not question. Questions and concerns are not part of the Vision Statement or Professional Policy Guidelines. It feels like a treadmill that can't stop.

For most of us, the sense of community we experienced in the past has all but disappeared. We live more time consuming hectic lives that do not afford us the time or energy to commit to community projects and activities.

Oh well, that's why we have communities, so others can do things for us, we muse. Who really is the community? The physical dividing lines between communities are disappearing as urban sprawl continues unabated. Where do we belong at all? Who do we relate with? Someone tells us we live in a global community. What does this mean? At best we know only a few members of our immediate community anyway. Isolation, resentment and fear continue to set in. We have a blurred sense that life isn't working.

This is a sample of our moment-to-moment, day-after-day, year-after-year struggle. As years go by, external circumstances change, but the inner struggle continues creating the same outer life. We have survived but call it living. Nothing changes and we are exhausted! This is our life!

# Chapter 2
# *What Do We Want?*

What is it most of us are seeking? What do we want? Or do we ever reflect on this? Surely we have given up so much in exchange for the turmoil of our lives. Most likely we might say we are seeking happiness and inner peace. We want a sense of security from a world that is ridden with strife. Possibly we want to love, be loved, enjoy ourselves and be part of a community. We want a sense that we are part of the solution in the world.

How do we go about this? The lives we have created and live each day don't really give us these things. We have convinced ourselves that they do. We are easily caught in what everyone else seems to be doing and telling us. Our lives have become the product of a snowball rolling down the hill getting larger and faster all the time. We barely see anything skim by as we barrel down the hill.

One distinction that must be made clear is the difference between gratification and happiness. Often we try to find happiness through gratification. We cannot *find* happiness. We cannot *seek* happiness. Happiness is a by-product or spin-off of something else. It *is* simply here. It *is* living life each moment the most appropriate way possible. It *is* our life. Unfortunately what we are usually seeking instead is gratification or pleasure. The experience of sensual enjoyment is involved. There is nothing wrong with pleasure. The act of eating a delicious ice cream cone is sensual. The taste and feel of the ice cream flowing over our tongue is exhilarating and enjoyable. But we soon want to repeat the experience to keep the pleasure endlessly alive. This in itself is not happiness.

In our quest for happiness we seek things that will give us a sense of permanence. We want the knowledge and feeling that we are safe and things will be the same tomorrow and the next day. So we continually repeat a list of pleasure seeking activities that we hope will bring us peace and happiness. It is comparable to eating more and more ice cream cones at a faster pace, so there is no time or space to look and see what is really happening. And so go our lives!

Our quest for happiness is often confused with the issue of avoiding physical or emotional pain. This notion is very much reinforced by the medical and mental health communities. To have physical pain in our bodies is perfectly normal because we are sentient beings. The author is not suggesting to deliberately cause harm to oneself so we can experience pain. That is foolish. We cannot escape the fact that biologically we are animals. If pain can be simply dealt with, then it is prudent to do so. But the relentless search for drugs and other treatments simply becomes the gratification of the endless ice cream cones. It is a distraction from facing life. Simply feel the pain and get on with life.

Similarly we have come to a place where we do not want emotional pain. But is this not part of life? Sometimes we must make difficult decisions, live with difficult situations and accept the consequences. Things happen that are perfectly part of life, even when they seem unpleasant. Accidents, death and so on are often difficult to deal with, but still are simply part of life. Somehow we have pushed them aside by living an isolated sterile image of life. We seem to confuse facing these issues with the continuous gratification of trying to escape them and inappropriately looking for answers. Sometimes we have to struggle in life. This is normal, this *is* life, and does not necessarily suggest an absence of happiness.

We live more instantaneously in today's world than ever before. We communicate around the world in microseconds. We play computer games that give us instant feedback without pause or reflection. We want things to happen faster and faster. This is a quality of instant sensual pleasure. It wasn't many years ago that to communicate with someone we wrote a letter and waited many days for a reply to arrive. In that time interval so many things could happen. There was anticipation, delaying gratification, anxiety, wondering what will be said, and so on. We had to wait, not knowing the outcome and not having the instant gratification. We had the time and space for more reflection and appropriate action.

Each of us deeply needs to know what we want and what is important. Not what we think we want or what society tells us we want. We must put tremendous energy into looking at this question. What we want can only be in the context of our relationship with everything. This is explored in the chapter on Relationship. When we have a clear notion of what we want, we command our lives. Otherwise we are being pulled in many directions by other forces. We still must make difficult choices and remain with the decisions. Jiddu Krishnamurti, a spiritual inspiration once stated, "Most of us want to have our cake and eat too. We do not want to give up a certain amusement-park attitude toward life."

We need to translate our wants into specific actions. One action for example might be to be a role model for our children and engage in many adventurous family activities. We now need to visualise what action that looks like. We require focused intention to bring about this goal of family adventure. What activities are planned, when, how are they organized? In summary it is knowing what we want, planning the specifics and executing the actions required. All this comes from a position of intention, or commitment.

Taisen Deshimaru Roshi asked, "Human beings are afraid of dying. They are always running after something: money, honour, pleasure. But if you had to die now, what would you want?" Find out!

# Chapter 3
# *Cultural Addiction*

Over time there have been countless cultures. Many factors such as geography, climate, technology, health, and religious views have contributed to their evolution. The differences in the cultures have been enormous. It is not the intention of the author to present an overview of various cultures but to refer to them in general where necessary.

Obviously if each of us lived in another culture we would experience a much different life. Technology, tools, geography and availability of food would have played an important role in how we lived. On more subtle levels clothing, religious views, social structure and so on would have defined how we lived. Yet we are human beings in both circumstances living very different lives.

The author does not deny variable genetic constitution as well as the interplay of genetics and environment. The complex tapestry between brain structure/ function and life as it is cannot be overlooked either. Nevertheless it is logical to suggest that we live different lives, with different expectations and values according to the culture we live in. Then what is it to be a whole, functioning human being when we remove the variable culture? Who are we really? How do we really behave? What do we want?

In the present culture of the Western World many of us are excited about the latest model of a particular car. If we could bring forth someone from a culture existing thousands of years ago and introduce him to the car we have no idea what his response might be. Nevertheless it may be safe to say there may be confusion and questioning as to what all the excitement is about. In addition he may show us a piece of silk and his donkey that are important to him. He may suggest his donkey is the best transportation possible. We may ask why the excitement about the donkey as transportation when we have this new car. We don't really understand each other. We live in different contexts.

Does this make someone right and someone wrong? Who is the whole human being? Maybe both, either or none. If either of us was transposed from one culture to the other, would we simply exchange behaviours to relate to the other culture? A good guess may be yes. After experiencing first hand the examples of each culture, the question becomes, does one have a choice as to what he really chooses to value? Can the author look at the donkey and the lifestyle it affords and decide to utilize it for transportation over the new car? That's more difficult to answer.

We all have examples of people in our lives that do behave to a varying degree outside the norms of our culture. But we need to be aware of the people who simply respond as rebels. This is simply the reaction of someone who has not inquired deeply within themselves and the relationship they have with the culture. An example of someone who chooses to live outside the norms of the culture might be someone who chooses not to own a car, which to a significant degree is a defining aspect of our culture. The person may well understand it is sometimes more convenient to a have a car but for reasons such as pollution or congestion chooses not to.

We have different cultures throughout the world at this very moment. In some ways they vary as much as cultures that existed long ago vary from us. Cultures of today vary in many aspects such as religion, language, work ethic, values, clothing and eating habits. To a great extent each of us has *chosen* to live the life more or less of one culture. We often suggest we were *born into* a particular culture or religion, and that is it. Many of us are now living more multicultural lives where we are blending aspects of various cultures. As well we also are attempting to hold onto some aspects of one culture while we integrate with others. It is quite obvious this life-style does not always support a life of harmonious relationships and simple flow.

We can be very cemented to our behaviour as defined by our culture. Take the simple example of eating. Persons of two cultures gather to eat. Immediately the questions of what to eat, how to eat it, and how to socialize around the process arise. What is really going on? We all require nourishment. Does it matter what and how it goes in? There seems to be some *other* dictating how we eat. Yet we give it such extraordinary importance. We continue to reinforce our polarized positions reflecting our cultural views.

The question becomes, why do we behave like this and is it necessary? This question can be extended to every aspect of our lives. Who is to say what is the correct way to worship and speak? Who is to say how to behave and dress, and what to value? The author is suggesting the question is about, "what it is to be human"? Then time and culture have less influence. Possibly we have much more freedom to choose our behaviour than imagined. As stated earlier, this does not deny the existence of brain structure/function, the relationship with the environment, and the role of genetics.

We were not born with a label adhering to our body saying we belong to this culture or that one. A baby is simply born of two human beings. Yes, there may be particular physical traits in the new-born suggesting a particular line of genetic endowment or culture as we know it. We may safely suggest that this group has a *history*. But it is only a story now. Nevertheless in our minds this suggests a closed group that now separates "us" from "others". We identify with it. That is us. Others are the others. Now we have the ongoing tension between "us" and "them". It can not stop as long as there is "me" and "them."

What happens when we attempt to trace back the the genetic and social structure of any particular culture? It becomes quite blurred. Other groups probably combined at different points in evolution as well as other interventions such as disease, floods and famine. It then becomes so blurred we simply do not know. We are not sure who belongs where. We still may have a story or theory, but it can only be very vague. It becomes more evident we are simply a species with individuals who have learned to behave in different fashions consistent with what surrounds us. We all have the common bond of being human beings and all that naturally goes with that.

A passage from the book *Call Girls* by Arthur Koestler seems relevant, "It seems to me that the disasters of our history are mainly due to our irresistible urge to become identified with a group, nation, church or what have you, and to espouse its beliefs uncritically and enthusiastically."

We are simply suggesting that our moment-to-moment daily lives are heavily regimented by our culture. The inner struggle to maintain ties to a culture creates the outer struggle of our lives. To suggest we want to make significant changes in our lives strongly implies that we step outside our cultural framework and the conditioning that has bound us. The only thing that keeps us there are beliefs.

# Chapter 4
# *Beliefs*

A man is walking along a path in the forest. He glances down and sees a poisonous snake on the path in front of him. Fearing for his life, he immediately removes his knife from it's sheath and aggressively begins to slice away at the snake. He does not stop until he is convinced it is dead and can not harm him. Slowly backing away while taking a deep breath he glances at the mutilated snake. What appears before him is a piece of discarded rope lying on the path. This is how most of us live our lives. We have little awareness.

Our moment-to-moment daily lives roll on as we feel trapped, helpless, thinking that we are saving the world, or believing others are responsible for our actions. There is no conscious personal world without thought and attached meaning. In other words, we have made everything up. Try it and see. When we shift our view everything changes. This leaves the fact that everything is conceptual. It is made up in our minds. Our world is what we believe it is. It is imagination. So what is left?

Remember our discussion regarding cultures? Our view/ behaviour of life appears to be influenced by our surroundings. Imagine we have no culture at all. We are born and raised in isolation. The author accepts the notion we require nurturing and support in surviving. But who are we and how do we behave? Unfortunately we are attracted to anything that is in front of us and accept it as truth. If our surroundings suggest we are an angel that is probably how we will behave. If our surroundings suggest we are a devil that is how we will behave. The truth in front of us remains undisturbed.

We have the conscious choice to do what we see fit. When we *see past* identifying with our surroundings we can afford any choice. If there is no conscious world without personal thought and meaning, what do we do? The exploration begins! Just observe. Extremely carefully watch the trees, flowers, birds, fish, animals, humans and so on. Just observe, remembering anything we think, imagine, label or believe is just made up in our heads. The incredible tapestry that the universe has sent us is all there. It operates the only way it can. Notice how beautiful and majestic each creation is. The tree for example is home to birds and insects. It emits oxygen to the air and supplies us with shade.

We can safely suggest the trees, animals and so on do not create stories and images of importance. They simply exist and have great importance to nature's equilibrium as previously stated. Then are we not obligated to do the same? Each creation comes from a position of nothing. It does not belong to a particular culture, or doesn't mean anything unless we give it meaning.

But we say we are educated, we have learned just about all things and have a handful of diplomas to prove it. We have been promoted to a level of responsibility and everyone around supports us. We have a Professional Policy and a Company Vision Statement. We have a fancy title on our office door. Wonderful, maybe it helps sometimes. But it does not change the absolute fact that we are operating from a position of nothing. Everything we think we have learned is simply that, we think, but we don't know. We believe.

We have chosen to live in a group and create something we have called a society. Next we have chosen to believe that our lives are created by society and we are a helpless product of that society. But each of us has created society by our behaviour and beliefs. Society is operating out of a position of nothing just as we are and following our misguided lives. When we see the truth of this we don't need to follow the expectations of society.

As long as we rigourously follow the expectations of society, the inner struggle continues to maintain identity with our personal integrity and society that each of us has created. This manifests in the outer moment-to-moment daily struggle of our lives. The rush, confusion, lack of enjoyment and applying inappropriate meaning continues. The author does not suggest we reject anything without rigourous observation. On the other hand all aspects of our individual and group behaviours are critically important. For example, we need to behave in orderly fashion while driving on the road. Everyone has equal importance and we will all get to our destinations when we wait for our turn, without being aggressive and threatening one another.

Our task is to acknowledge the things we cannot change and make informed decisions about what we can change. We need to rigourously question everything about ourselves and life. Yes, we say, but what will others think? We can't turn down a promotion, a raise, an invitation to join a particular group and so on. We will be outcasts, ridiculed. Remember that is a thought coming from nothing. All action is a conscious choice. It is simply a belief to think it is important to accept a promotion. We are free to choose and reap the benefits of life. We now have extraordinary space in which to live our lives. The people who don't choose appropriately don't reap the benefits, and live with stress.

The door to understanding this is to see the facts or truth, otherwise we are simply left with beliefs. Confusion and stress continue until we understand that life doesn't conform to our ideas about it. We have the conscious choice to do whatever, and we are absolutely responsible for each choice and the lives we live. Dr. David Bohm, a renowned physicist and observer of life, states it differently, "it is up to each individual to ask if I want to live the rest of my life playing out yet another variation of contemporary values? Am I willing to test the boundaries of my self-world view, in order to glimpse a larger, very different universe? Am I willing to take risks for the possibility of new understanding, knowing there can be no money-back guarantee?"

# Chapter 5

# *Awareness*

If only for a fleeting moment we can put aside the sense we think we know something and just wonder, we have made huge leaps. We were positive what Aunt Jean meant by that statement. Now we are not sure, she might have meant several different things. How do we remain open to the limitless possibilities of each moment? Part of the notion of beliefs is assumptions. I know the company will deliver the product I ordered today because they said they would. We don't know! They simply said they would. I may receive it or I may not. Being addicted to the assumption I will receive it brings the possibility of grief. When we are open to all possibilities there are no surprises. Then we deal with the situation.

The Oxford Dictionary defines the word *perception* as: "the intuitive recognition of a truth, an interpretation or impression based on one's understanding of something ...." In other words, it is how each of us views ourselves, the events in our life, and the world in general. It is how each of us translates all of our life experiences into meaning. Our awareness is the outcome of our perception. Perception becomes a learned act of constructing reality to fit one's assumption about it. Each of us is believed to develop a restricted set of perceptions through our own unique transactions with the environment.

Perception is a learned act, and how we perceive something determines our attitude towards it. Our perception is our individual frame of reference about life, love, reality, along with our values and attitudes. Put differently, the depth to which we see the truth of a situation is controlled by our past experiences, interpretations, and beliefs. Each of us has built our own unique framework that encloses the process of creating our perception. We are boxed in by the process used to create it, as well as our perception itself, and can't see beyond it. This becomes our level of awareness.

There are some things we can do or be aware of to improve the accuracy of our level of perception. Those of us who feel comfortable with life and carry healthy self-esteem respond to situations differently from those who feel alienated or hostile. We adapt to life differently therefore interpret it differently. Those of us who trust life and what it has to offer process our experiences differently. Our physical health is a factor in determining how we see and interpret the world. Our individual goals and values influence how we see life.

Question everyone and everything very deeply! This may appear to be difficult. Most of us have a forbidden list of people or organizations that we do not question. The list may include our doctor, lawyer, mental health professional, educator, religious leader, and so on. If anything, we should give more attention to questioning the people on our forbidden list than others. Those are the ones we most likely have followed in a blind fashion. This does not mean we rudely and openly challenge everything said. But we quietly and firmly doubt everything, and probe deeply.

Bring a sense of wonder to each moment and what people are suggesting. Remember no matter what training or experience someone has had they are simply a product of their culture, training, beliefs, awareness, personality traits, ego and so on. We need to simply see people and their situations as they are. This attitude and skill often takes considerable practice. When we cultivate this practice in our moment-to-moment lives we are left with little room for surprises.

How are we aware of anything? We are aware through the response to a stimulus. When we touch a hot stove we know first hand what it feels like. We learn quickly through identification whether this is a pleasurable activity or a painful one. As discussed previously we decide to repeat the pleasurable, gratifying experiences. On the other hand we learn to avoid painful experiences. We have drawn conclusions about the world by identifying with these two qualities. This is not bad in itself. Using the example of the stove, it is prudent to be careful around hot stoves.

We have converged our existence to the repetition of pleasurable experiences and the avoidance of physical and emotional painful ones. The complete constellation of our daily activities is under this umbrella. We are not aware that almost everything we do and don't do is restricted by our seeking pleasure and avoiding pain. No wonder we feel unhappy, pressured and stressed. We are continually eating the sensual ice cream cones, then trying to avoid the pain of the weight gain. Another example is working long hours at a job doing things we don't enjoy, while questioning the ethical issues involved. All this is to avoid the perception we are financially falling behind our peers.

To cultivate our awareness we must step outside our pain-pleasure activities. To do so we must first be acutely aware how the pain-pleasure issue operates in our lives. When we receive the visual stimulus of a new car we immediately have a pleasurable identity with it. We continuously desire the car, reinforcing the pleasure seeking of the brain. We eventually go to any lengths to obtain the car and put ourselves under financial strain, or whatever else to obtain it. Once we get the car we have our antenna out because the pleasure is wearing off and we require another fix. It is an endless cycle. When we observe this cycle in ourselves we see the futility of it. We make appropriate changes to step outside of it. We tell ourselves to stop this.

There is an old saying, "the more I think I know, the more I realize I don't know." The same can be said about awareness. The more aware we become, the more we realize we are not aware at all. In other words our lives can change dramatically and quickly when we see that what we have felt or thought has little or no reality base. We just thought it did.

This leaves a huge emptiness to fill with the facts. In our example of the car, we realize that we did not need it we just identified with the sensual pleasures of being present with it. We are now content to drive our old rusty car. It does not make it wrong to have a new car, we just must be clear why we have one. Put another way, a change in meaning is a change in being. In all areas of our lives this takes vigilance. A whole new way of being is present when we realize things are not as they appear.

# Chapter 6
# *Thoughts and Feelings*

Our moment-to-moment, day-to-day lives are filled with a constant flood of feelings. Feelings of frustration, anger, depression, joy, and so on dominate our existence. Our behaviour of rushing, pleasing, not paying attention, and so on then becomes an outcome of these feelings. We have put so much emphasis on feelings and reacting to them, trying to control or abolish them. Our lives seem to be out of control because we are trying to control the wrong things. When we are feeling upset and sad we find we can't simply will ourselves into living meaningfully. Are we really aware of what is going on?

Feelings and thoughts act in similar ways. They continuously rise. It is our job to see this and deal with it. They may or may not have any particular meaning or importance. They speak for themselves. If something is to be learned, then do so. Suffice it to say that it is prudent to simply see most thoughts and feelings as something to let go as they rise. But we have a practice of holding on to them and making far too much meaning out of them. There is little need to dissect them, or attempt to abolish them. Can we simply accept feelings and emotional reactions to events as they are?

David Reynolds in his book *Constructive Living* outlines five principles in better understanding how feelings affect our lives:

• Feelings are uncontrollable directly by the will.

In other words we can't make ourselves feel anything. We can't think or feel our way out of them.

• Feelings must be recognized and accepted as they are.

If we can't think or feel our way out of them then the best strategy is to accept them and see what we can learn from them. Sometimes feelings give us clues about something we need to do. In this case we are responsible to do what needs to be done. For example if someone is anxious about not having homework done, it may be wise to do the homework. In this case the feelings will now change.

• Every feeling, however unpleasant, has its uses.

Grief prompts revaluation and a change in behaviour; anxiety leads to care and preparation; guilt causes to us to re-examine; fear mobilizes our bodies for action. Within the most unpleasant emotions there is potential for good. Realizing this there is no scurrying to avoid them.

• Feelings fade in time unless they are re-stimulated.

Given time the worst scenarios change, lose their edge or become little more than a memory. This principal applies to pleasant feelings as well. The joy of this moment will soon fade. Our feelings can be revitalized by numerous events such as a movie, an argument, a discussion and so on.

• Feelings can be indirectly influenced by behaviour.

This is the gold nugget in the pot! We can use our behaviour to bring about desirable feelings, and reduce the influence of undesirable ones. This is the handle on our feelings that life has graciously supplied to us. For example, Jennifer feels depressed about being overweight. She needs to eat less and exercise more. But she is not in the mood and only complains. In other words she lets her feelings control her behaviour and the result is more depression. The reality is Jennifer must intervene herself, and change her eating/exercise pattern. Then her feelings will change. Obviously certain strong feelings are intransigent and are not easily affected by our behaviour. They must wane under principal four.

We all struggle in non-productive ways because we don't see how these principals work in our lives. They are nothing more than common-sense observations. We can deal with continually rising thoughts in a similar manner. The result being the more we release thoughts and feelings and control our actions the more empowered we are in our lives. The more empowered we are the less stress we experience. This leads to the critical point: We are responsible for what we do no matter how we feel at the time.

Lets face it, emotion is an intrinsic evolutionary response aimed at self-preservation. The key is to use our emotions to our advantage. If needed, we turn them into anger and then focus. These are deliberate actions. We are now prepared to do what needs to be done each moment. To live appropriately though, we need to balance emotion with reason.

All of us have used an endless list of excuses for behaving irresponsibly: I didn't feel like it, I was upset, I was tired, I was scared, and so on. In each case though, we have control over the action of choice. Sometimes we may have to exert ourselves, and it may not be easy. The result is possibly  slipping back into the pattern of letting our feelings control our behaviour. It may appear that being responsible for our actions is a boring life, where all we do is be responsible.

But this is the very point! It is these times when we create order, feel most in control and responsible in our lives, that we feel most free. It appears paradoxical. We are then free to feel a whole range of emotions that we did not before. This in turn allows us to enjoy many more  activities. The process continues. Remember, it begins with a firm grip on our behaviour without the excuses.

Ordered, constructed behaviour can also be used to create feelings that we desire. We can create a hyped-up feeling by dancing, running, sports, listening to music, having a provocative conversation, and so on. Similarly we can create a calming feeling by listening to soothing music, having a massage, practising yoga, and so on. We can create many moods we want on a daily basis by choosing our actions. When we observe our lives we might notice the times of greatest reward and satisfaction were those when we accomplished something or completed a goal when inner and outer obstacles were great. But we maintained our focus on our behaviour, not our feelings and thoughts.

Many years ago Plato stated, "emotions can trump reason, so in order to succeed we have to use the reins of reason on the horse of emotion."

# Chapter 7
# *What Is Stress?*

Most of us have experienced what we view as stress in our lives. We feel rushed and are not doing the things we think are important. We are not spending enough time with our families, not enjoying our avocations, feeling pushed to meet the demands of a boss, and more. The effects of stress show up as emotional and physical manifestations. We are irritable, more sensitive, and ill more often.

The word *stress* means different things to different people so we require a common understanding in order to look at the topic. The surgeon about to begin an operation is under stress. The business person continually trying to please clients, create more sales, and get recognized is under stress. The person who is ill in bed is under stress. The person driving the car  trying to avoid an accident is under stress. Each of us is under stress while breathing polluted air. The individual held at gun point during a robbery is under stress. The athlete standing on the starting line of the world championship marathon race is under stress. The situations are different for each, but stress is present.

The stress producing factors, called *stressors* are different yet the body reacts in similar fashion to each. The reactions may include such things as rapid heart beat, sweating, anxious feelings, blurred awareness, and so on. There is a clear distinction between stress and stressors. One is the result of the other. On one hand putting forth the desire and effort to win the world marathoning championship may be worth the stress involved. It may even be a stress we desire, knowing we need it to be successful. We know the stress is time limited (the perception of control). However if the stress is too much we reduce our chances of winning. On the other hand undergoing the stress of a gun point robbery may not be the stress of choice. We don't know if we will live, how long it will last, and there is nothing for us to gain by it (the perception of little control).

In other words we generally want to avoid the bad effects of stress, and enjoy the pleasurable by-products it has to offer. Seems fair enough, but we can't have it all ways. If we want to create or complete something we require a certain amount of stress whether we like it or not, like the athlete ready to perform. The effect of stress is the effect of stress no matter what kind.

One way we might define stress is: the biological and/or the psychological response of the body to any demand made upon it. Put another way we might refer to it as the reaction we have to a situation where we believe our well being is endangered or threatened in some way. For the sake of discussion we can divide stress into two categories. *Distress* might be described as the unwanted reaction to a certain situation such as a gun point robbery. The stress that we invite when we want to optimize maximum performance is called *eustress*. Examples of this might be the surgeon ready to operate, or the athlete ready to perform.

The same biochemical changes occur in the body whether we experience eustress or distress. These changes have quite specific effects on the body. It is not the intent of the author to describe in any detail what changes take place. Except to say that the body releases excessive amounts of corticoid hormones that have negative effects on our health, both short and long term. As well, there can be significant emotional outcomes. The effects of both eustress and distress are cumulative.

In summary, as suggested earlier it appears that we perform optimally under a certain amount of stress, such as the athlete ready to perform. But excessive stress inhibits performance. Stress is not all bad. We need a certain amount in our lives. The issue seems to be more about questions such as:

• do we perceive a sense of control in the situation?

• what types of stressors are involved?

• what quantity of stressors are involved?

• for how long are we exposed to the stressors?

• how aware are we of our individual natural temperament?

• what coping mechanisms have we developed over the span of our lives?

• how aware are we of our level of resilience and hardiness in life?

• what is our general world view?

Obviously the effect of stressors is very personal and variable. Any two people in similar circumstances may report widely varying views and reactions. So the issue is more about getting to know ourselves better, watching how we react in different situations and developing alternate coping techniques. This is built on our awareness of topics discussed earlier such as cultural addiction, beliefs, a sense of what is *really* going on and clearly prioritizing what we want in life. Each of us is responsible for tailor making coping strategies that best suit our individual needs.

While walking in the woods we are confronted by an

angry brown bear and immediately feel afraid, and rightly so. Adrenaline as well as other steroids are quickly circulating through the body. Our heart rate increases. Possibly our muscles feel frozen. We are feeling stressed. Our lives are in danger. The sooner we relieve ourselves of the situation the safer we will feel and our stress level will return to normal (whatever that is for each of us). This stressor is time limited. We either get away quickly or it is too late.

This type of stress we might call *acute* stress. It lasts for a relatively short period of time and can be intense. Because it is of short duration the bodily functions quickly return to normal and we are on our merry way. No harm done. Other examples might be car accidents, listening to a boring speech, or being temporarily unemployed. Many of these situations are unavoidable. They are simply part of life.

We may avoid most of them if we live our lives in a closet, but that really isn't living. So we must simply view them as part of the price of being alive. It is short term because we are exposed for a specific time frame, and won't have to deal with them after the incident is over. In a few situations people have lingering effects after episodes of acute stress. This often appears to result from unrealistic world views, low self-esteem or inappropriate coping skills.

On the other hand, the second general type of stress is more subtle, long lasting and can have devastating physical and emotional effects on us. This we might call *chronic* stress. An example might be looking after a critically ill family member for a long period of time. In this case there is no relief, there is emotional strain, the body is stressed with lack of sleep and nourishment, there is no apparent time frame for ending, and there exists a general feeling of having little control in life. There is little opportunity to refocus, or do something else we might want to do. Our reaction to chronic stress seems to be the area were we experience significant difficulty. Adrenaline and other steroids circulate through the body indefinitely and take their toll emotionally and physically.

There appears to be no let up. Other examples of chronic stress might be working in a job we do not enjoy, or being continually verbally or physically abused.

Coping styles for chronic stress differ depending on the psychological make-up of the individual involved. For example the stress experienced by a surgeon working long, continuous hours yet loving his work might be handled differently than the stress experienced by someone living in financial strain. No matter what, the body experiences the *fight or flight response.* In the case of acute stress of the bear attacking we have the choice of fighting or fleeing. Whichever choice we make let's assume it was the correct one. The point being we have returned to a position of safety and the body's defence mechanism has returned to normal. The body is biologically designed to operate in the fight or flight mode. The stress has a short time duration and comes to a resolution.

The difficulty sets in with chronic stress. We often cannot deal with a situation using the natural fight or flight mechanism. A person in a job with unrealistic expectations, long hours and a miserable boss may not be able to use the fight or flight response. Yes, we can fight with the boss but this might not be the most prudent choice. We may not be able to flee the job if we require the income. But it might be wise to look long term at fleeing. This entails planning for other income sources, and finding the resources to leave the job sometime in the future. This is an example of appropriate stress management. But if we do not take action with the situation then we are under long-term stress, which takes its toll. When there is little action we can take, we need to look more closely at changing our attitude, such as the case of prisoners of war. Put simply, we need appropriate planning and action, and then the fight or flight response takes its course.

## Emotional Symptoms of Stress

• depression • anxiety • aggression • lack of feeling

in control • feelings of helplessness • despair • changes in motivation • irritability • fatigue • lethargy • changes in sleep pattern • withdrawn • being argumentative • changes in participation with hobbies • don't have time • blaming • projecting • changes in drug/alcohol use • changes in eating habits • changes in weight • changes from healthy personal boundaries • not enjoying relationships • changes in levels of responsibility for our actions • changes in spending habits • changes in personal care/grooming • changes in judgement • changes in short and long term planning habits • changes in enthusiasm • always wanting to get ahead • excessive self focus • not seeing "the humour" of a situation • changes in sense of gratitude • changes in amount of energy spent looking outside ourselves for answers

This list is not conclusive. It is a guideline that can be considered when we or others notice at least several factors have changed over a significant duration of time. We all might experience many of these symptoms on a daily basis just because of the nature of our lives. But they generally do not continue, or become chronic. We are more concerned with longer term changes that suggest distress. It is important to understand the changes are personal and relative to each individual. We all have different base lines of behaviour and coping mechanisms. So we must be aware of the changes relative for an individual and not attempt to compare changes with someone else. They have a whole different constellation of strengths, weaknesses, coping mechanisms, natural tendencies and more, than we do.

## Physical Symptoms of Stress

• tight muscles • general physical tension • increased heart rate • increased blood pressure • increase in blood sugar • eye tension • dilated pupils • frowning • shallow breathing • poor sleeping habits • increased perspiration • manual dexterity changes • difficulty focusing on tasks • changes in libido • slurred speech • hurrying • constant colds, flu, etc. • nausea

• dry mouth • irritable bowel/bladder • physical symptoms unexplained by physician • obsessive/compulsive behaviour • weight gain/loss

Again this list is not conclusive and individually each symptom is not necessarily stress-related. We are looking for patterns of numerous symptoms observed over significant time. These are to be correlated with other factors. There is significant medical literature suggesting a relationship between stress and major serious chronic illnesses.

# Chapter 8
# *Coping*

The feeling or thought that our lives are out of control induces the stress response mechanism in the body. The surgeon working with precision cannot make a mistake. The marathon runner attempting to win the world championship places stress on himself. Over time the effects of stress could kill these people. But it doesn't. In many examples a brief period of exposure (often longer) to stress can be beneficial. In other words the surgeon requires the stress of being perfect in order to successfully complete the operation. He could not have done it without the stress. He has adapted to the requirements of the situation. The marathon runner adapts to the demands of the race. It's when we feel our lives are out of control we may experience some of the symptoms discussed earlier. But we get by. How? We have adapted to a situation. We might define *adaptation* as ability to fit, modify or alter.

This is a crucial point to understand. We all have the ability to adapt to situations we have never been in, or ones we think we could never survive. An example of the body adapting is a distance runner putting more demands of speed and endurance than ever on the body. Continuing to do this over a period of time, the runner is now capable of much more with less difficulty.

Similarly we have the psychological/emotional ability to adapt to different situations. Returning to the example of the gun point robbery, we might feel scared, angry and so on yet at some level there might be confidence and assurance we will survive. In some way we have adapted to the situation even if we didn't like it. If we notice, the incident may have expanded our sense of confidence to better cope with future unpleasant events.

Each of us has created a mental map of what life is, and what it should be. This is based on our past experience. But reality this moment is invariably different from our map. The greater the distance between our mental map and reality, the greater our difficulty coping. The mind wants to live in it's mental map or story about how life should be. The sooner we accept reality as it is now, the sooner we create a new mental map. Then we have little difficulty coping because our new map resonates with reality. Now we have literally become a different person. The old one has gone. We have found our true self which is only synchronization with this true moment. Notice, in your own life, the times you felt better when you accepted a situation. It doesn't mean you had to like it.

We are also talking about a sense of *resilience* which might be described as the ability to recoil, rebound or have a sense of elasticity. In other words, after a stressful situation we return to a state of *homeostasis* or the condition we were previously in. Physically and emotionally we are like elastics. The elastic has a resting position which is equivalent to our everyday level of stress where we do quite well. The elastic expands to larger sizes by the stress of being pulled and returns to normal size after the stress is released. No harm is done. This is very comparable to a human being reacting to a stressor. But we have much more room to stretch and cope than we realize. Let's look at times in our lives when we stretched and survived but thought we were not going to. Now we know that in the future we have so much more space in which to allow ourselves to cope.

Yes, when pulled too hard the elastic breaks. It does not return to its normal position. It can not serve its previous function. The same is true for each of us. We reach a breaking point and physically and/or emotionally break. We can no longer function in the previous ways and require specific help and time to heal, if indeed we do. The breaking point is much further away for each of us than we realize. We have assumed or created beliefs that we can't cope, or we have never tested ourselves to find out. Often we let fear take over in a situation, then our old beliefs take over again. Let's look for examples of this in our lives. This cannot be emphasised enough ... we have so much resiliency and ability to adapt in order to get by.

Our task is to understand ourselves better. Each of is capable of adapting and coping to different extents. The reasons are numerous. We are all born with different innate temperaments. We have a lifetime of experiences we have interpreted and made into stories. We have our unique self-image. We are each faced with the task of understanding our strengths, weakness and current coping mechanisms. Only then can we realistically evaluate how and to what extent we can cope in particular situations. It is then our responsibility to live within the bounds of our understanding. In other words we are responsible for creating our lives within the context of knowing ourselves. This is a unique individual task for each of us. No one can give us a formula for doing this.

Studies suggest that individuals demonstrating characteristics of *hardiness* show less stress related symptoms and are less likely to become ill after significantly stressful events. Hardiness might be considered as being made up of three components: commitment, control and challenge. *Commitment* is the willingness to be completely involved in a task. *Control* is the attitude that we are empowered and can influence the world by our actions. *Challenge* means we understand that change is ongoing and natural. We see it as the spice of life. Look carefully in yourself for these three components.

As we know life presents us with situations that are different or more painful than we have ever experienced before. We feel we have no background or experience for dealing with a particular situation. Examples of this might be the death of a loved one, the loss of all our possessions during a hurricane or being told we have a terminal illness. Yet we are being asked to cope the best we can with these developments. We are entering a new territory of life. We will be asking fundamental questions to ourselves such as what is the meaning of life, of suffering, why me, why should I go on. On the surface this is a natural thing to be doing. It is the process of coping and making sense out of our world. It is not intended to be easy. But it is our task to find our way using whatever means possible, and not to look for someone to save us, because they can't.

Wonderful examples of coping might be taken from the book *Man's Search for Meaning* by Dr. Viktor Frankl. Viktor was a psychiatrist who recounts his experiences in a German prisoner of war camp during WW2. He describes the most brutal living conditions possible to imagine. Men were regularly put on the train and sent to the gas chambers. If one was fortunate enough to escape that fate, daily life was reduced to its most naked form. Many men died in the camp from the physical and/or emotional nature of the experience. Starvation, beatings, and winter work camps with little clothing were the daily routine. Viktor (obviously himself a survivor) noticed that there were common qualities among those who survived:

• each person endured much more than they ever believed possible.

• when stripped of all the necessities of life there still remained the most important of all freedoms - the ability to "choose one's attitude in a given set of circumstances."

• in some fashion, by choosing to be "worthy of their suffering," they were able to rise above their outward fate.

• no matter what the circumstances each of them had a choice of action.

- those who had a reason to live found a way to live; for example to reunite with family or complete projects that were started before the war began.

- accepting that suffering is an ineradicable part of life.

In his book Viktor discusses what he viewed as reaching a pivotal point in his survival. He let go of his fear of dying. This does not mean he gave up or gave in to the guards. In fact, it meant quite the opposite. It just meant he wasn't attached to the outcome of wanting to live. He realized he probably would die, most were dying, that was the fact. So all that was important was this moment being alive. He then spent more time and effort trying to comfort other prisoners, giving them encouragement and sharing his food (crumbs of bread). This attitude and behaviour was frowned upon by the guards so brought Viktor more discomfort in some ways, and on the other hand he was seen as special and given extra privileges. He was more alive than ever. He was saying to himself and his peers that we may well die, so let's accept that and go down with a fight. Accepting his probable fate allowed him greater space to do what was needed.

This implication is very important to each of us. Whether in an uncomfortable position with our boss, family members or under financial strain the point is the same. We must accurately accept the reality of the situation and be prepared to accept the natural consequences. Then fight. There is no choice. If we identify with the fear of whatever may happen in the future, and let go of that ... it is only a possibility at this moment anyway ... we are free to engage all our energy and resources in dealing with the issue now. The result will be whatever it will be, but in the mean time we are dealing with what we can control now. It helps to keep in mind that each of us will meet  the same fate ... death ... the same fate the prisoners were trying to avoid. So yes, we can deal with anything!

Viktor Frankl went on to state that what was needed was a fundamental change in attitude towards life. *It did not really matter what we expected from life, but rather what life expected from us.* How simple and profound to make a shift from that point of reference. After all, expecting life to conform to our whims suggests each of us is the centre of the universe. Absolutely not! Obviously we are part of and responsible for something much larger and more profound than ourselves. It is our responsibility to function each moment within that context no matter what the external circumstances.

Few of us are living in such extreme situations as these men. So surely each of us can make choices of *attitude* and *action* in our everyday life that enables us to better cope. No matter how busy or frustrating our day is we can better deal with it. The six observations summarized from Viktor's book can be applied to our own everyday life. A problem is we often don't see the urgency to change our attitude and actions. But life is this moment for us just as it was each moment surviving in the concentration camp. Now is the moment of changing our life. There is an urgency! As in the concentration camp no one is coming to save us.

A simple example might be sitting in a traffic jam. Our usual reaction might be one of feeling out of control, angry, frustrated and knowing we will miss the meeting. If we pause and reflect on Viktor's observations we realise that right now, this is the reality of living in the city. We know we will physically survive. We realise we can endure much more than we think we can; for example we can be late, miss the meeting, and deal with any consequences. In other words we just change our attitude. Also, we have the choice to plan now to move to a different geographical location in the future.

In any situation, whether the work place, home or caring for an ill loved one, the task is the same: be orderly and methodical, set small obtainable goals, take responsibility, and focus. An example of a small obtainable goal might be to successfully get the patient to take their medication. When complete we move on to the next small obtainable goal. Ultimately it is the struggle that keeps one alive. What seems a paradox is simply the act of living. Life itself is a paradox, gathering order out of chaos.

This is what we must do. Then the very nature of life changes and we experience life differently. In his book *Deep Survival,* Laurence Gonzales states, " a survival situation (coping, stress) brings out the true underlying personality. Our survival kit is inside us. But unless it is there before called upon, it is not going to appear magically at the moment it is needed. When you consolidate your personality as a survivor, what you get is the essence of what you always had."

There is an interesting observation regarding being influenced by our surroundings/culture as discussed earlier. On one hand it is difficult to believe that the German soldiers would treat other human beings the way they did. In most cases they actually believed that it was appropriate. They had been under the influence of the Nazi propaganda machine for some time. It may be safe to assume they were raised in a fashion similar to how we were, with a variety of views on values, morals, family life and appropriate behaviour (whatever that is). Yet with a dangerous blend of surroundings and beliefs, they changed into who they were.

As discussed earlier in the chapters titled Cultural Addiction and Beliefs, it is obvious each of us is, to a great extent, our culture and our beliefs. This then does not remove us far from the behaviour of the soldiers. The point being, if we don't step outside our culture and beliefs and look at REALITY and take responsibility for our actions, then each of us is the same as the soldiers. Do we begin to see why the world is what it is? It is interesting to observe how many of us complain about the stressful meaningless lives we live. Does one not begin to wonder?

Generally there are three styles for coping with stressful events:

### • Task-Orientated Response

We analyse the situation and try to figure out what actions can be taken to deal directly with the problem.

### • Distraction-Orientated Response

We use recreational activities or hobbies to take our mind off the situation. Exercise is always beneficial because it helps the body clear away the toxins that are created by anxiety.

### • Emotion-Orientated Response

We focus on our feelings and find social supports to talk about them. Some individuals find comfort in talking about their concerns and hearing that they are shared. Others may find that their anxiety escalates as they discuss the situation and prefer to avoid talking directly.

It is the responsibility of each of us to determine the most adaptive way to cope. We all respond differently to stressful situations, and develop different coping strategies.

Long before our time Epictetus wrote, "on occasion of every event that befalls you, remember to turn to yourself and inquire as to what power you have for turning it to use."

# Chapter 9
# *Gratitude*

Lets return to the concentration camp for a moment. When the prisoners who had a survivor personality were given even the smallest piece of bread, or had one pea in the water they called soup, they were entirely grateful. They at least had a mouthful of food that day. If they made it to the end of the day without being beaten or even worse sent to the gas chamber, they were grateful. Most of us wouldn't imagine being grateful at all in this situation. Life is lived within a context. Obviously the prisoners were not concerned with fashionable clothes, fancy meals, cars, investments, getting promoted and so on. They wanted only to survive. Anything that supported the notion of survival was appreciated. Anything else was unnecessary to them.

Somewhere between this scenario and the lives most of us live today we seem to have lost our sense of life. To the prisoner each moment **is** life right now. Whether it was unpleasant, unfair, and so on is not the issue. Being stripped naked both physically and emotionally, they were taken to the core of life. They were thankful for anything that sustained them. Each of us also has that same naked core of life (whatever that might be). This is all we really need ... we are alive ... plus we have food, clothing, shelter, the appearance of safety and so on. We may not be doing exactly what we would choose to do right now but in the next moment we can create something else. Or in the case of the prisoners where their choices of action were limited, they were still free to choose their attitude, which sustained them.

We seemed to have covered over that naked core of life with many layers of material possessions, jobs, beliefs, theories, images, general busyness, and continually trying to better fit into the culture we have created, which in turn is our very downfall. Lets be clear on who has done this ... each of us ... not our culture, or someone else. Each of us is completely responsible for the lives we live right now. If each of us is not, then who is?

We have so much compared to the prisoners (using them as an example) and yet we feel, act and behave in a manner that suggests we don't have enough, and we are not happy. We simply need to turn our point of reference from what we don't have, to being thankful for what we do have. We need to change the context of our lives. Said differently, we need to inquire into the question, "what is it to be human?" We waste so much time and energy wishing for something that does not exist. Once our lives are over we cannot get them back no matter what we have or don't have. Each moment **is** life for each of us.

Many of us have noticed times in our own lives when we didn't really appreciate something until it was gone. An opportunity to be grateful was lost and we replaced it with another opportunity to be disappointed. Gratitude is something that is not necessarily controlled by our will. It requires some effort to begin. We need to pay attention and reflect. We need to notice the countless gifts, blessings and opportunities we are afforded each moment. The simple example of someone holding a door open for us is an extraordinary gift. When reflecting on what is happening we change the flow of our lives. We move from living in our heads concerned about what is wrong, to living moment-to-moment in our lives. Soon experiencing gratitude becomes self-sustaining. There is no alternative.

We tend to have an ideal of what life should be in particular situations. We then spend our energy trying to reach or create the image of the ideal. Of course this can rarely be done. Let's say tonight we want to have the most incredible dinner, created with the most exotic dishes from around the world and supplemented with the finest wines (the ideal). There is nothing wrong with this wish list for dinner, sounds great! For a variety of reasons it is probably not going to happen tonight. Immediately we are disappointed and frustrated. But if we attend to what is in the refrigerator and find some fresh vegetables, left over meat, fresh pasta and half a bottle of inexpensive wine opened yesterday we can make a great meal, be nourished and enjoy it. Not the ideal that we wanted but it fits reality at this moment. We appreciate the meal we made. We don't compare it to what might have been. That is something our mind made up. It does not exist, only reality exists.

This view can be applied to any situation in life. Whether it is our job, financial situation, family life, avocations and so on, our task is to recognize the ideals (images) we have created in our minds, but then act from a position of reality. We are then immediately grateful for what reality has given us. The recognition of how the mind looks for an ideal state is the critical first stage in opening ourselves to the gifts of life. Only the most arrogant among us can suggest what life should truly be.

When we expand our view and look at what life is offering, we notice we are surrounded by enormous support and love. We have everything we need, plus some. The more we are aware of life's gifts the more consistently we are open to receive more. In his book *Naikan Gratitude, Grace, and the Art of Self-Reflection,* author Gregg Krech suggests we ask ourselves three questions on a daily basis:

• what did I receive from others today?

• what did I give to others today?

• what troubles and difficulties did I cause others today?

There begins to emerge a completely different way of seeing life. We see we are not independent beings living independent lives. There is more of a sense of **us,** not just me. Life is a complex tapestry of interactions involving everyone.

Another exercise one might consider each evening is asking ourselves what we are grateful for that day. The exercise may seem difficult at first so try to choose several more obvious responses like, "I had food to eat today." As time passes try to lengthen the list and look for more subtle answers. An additional exercise might be asking ourselves what objects we are thankful for? Examples of responses to reflect on might be furnace, hat, coffee mug.

A further practice we might consider is, to go out of our way to thank someone for something they did for us. We may not usually thank the person who actually cooks the meal in the restaurant. But ask to speak to that person and thank them personally for the gift of our delicious meal. Look on a regular basis for opportunities to do this. This creates a shift in our attention each time we are thankful. We move away from a life of self-focus, towards a concern for others. They are us too. We change our very experience of life.

# Chapter 10
# *Creating Our Lives*

Most of us have heard the old saying that goes something like, change the things that need changing and accept the things we cannot change. Sometimes it appears difficult. Nevertheless it is the cornerstone of being in control of our lives, and living with less stress. If each of us doesn't take charge of our life, who will? Situations such as critical illness, death, divorce, loosing a job and so on often seem difficult to accept. Certainly often they are. Nevertheless there is no choice, we must. **This is the very task life is asking of us**.

The most remarkable human beings accept what they cannot change and at the same time empower themselves with things they can change. There is no one way of obtaining this essence. Often those of us who have been challenged repeatedly and to great depths have sorted out these qualities live meaningful, enjoyable lives. It is interesting to note that these are the people the rest of us often look toward and suggest that life is so easy for them, and say I wish I could be like that. The truth is they have created their life independent of the way things are, or has happened. That is the only difference.

This is our task ... to create our life with what we have at this moment. This may seem a bit out of sorts. We may respond with something like, "life is what has happened to me, it is awful". Well, yes and no! Things have happened that are unarguable and irrevocable. But we now have our choices to respond and act in the most empowered and responsible manner.

This opportunity changes our very experience of life and who we are now, absolutely in charge. This is a critical point. We may not have all the options we wish for just as the prisoners of war didn't. It may be comparable to a card game where we can only play with the cards we are dealt. We may pine for a card we don't have but that simply defers the game, drains energy and wastes time in constructing the next move with the cards in hand. It is the most arrogant and stupid among us who want to play with cards we simply don't have.

Al Siebert in his book *The Survivor Personality* writes," the best survivors (those who best cope) spend almost no time, especially in emergency situations, getting upset about what has been lost, or feeling distressed about things going badly ... for this reason they don't usually take themselves too seriously and are therefore hard to threaten."

A meaningful question in creating our life might be, why am I doing this right now? If this question can be reasonably answered, then we are engaged in reality dealing with life this moment, doing what can be done. It is the opposite of aimless moments, or blaming. It is the opposite of reacting from feelings, thoughts, philosophies, which only create further problems. The thrust is on doing, action, behaviour that is goal-directed (making appropriate changes, taking charge) and just observing feelings, not acting on them except when appropriate.

Very often the most miserable, ineffective people are ones who are feeling -orientated. They feel trapped and suggest they are victims. Life has done this or that to them. No wonder they feel stressed. Their energy is spent trying to change or reduce their feelings, creating even further distress. This process distracts them from what needs to be done immediately. In most cases using feelings as a barometer to evaluate our life is inappropriate.

But when the emphasis is on the task and not on ourselves an enormous transition occurs. What needs to be done is getting done. The importance of this switch in strategy cannot be over emphasised. We need to be aware of times we respond without observing, planning and acting. Then we develop the skill of using these three actions when dealing with a  particular situation. The more we practice this the more honed the skill becomes.

This is not to suggest that we should not be sensitive individuals with acute awareness of feelings. On the contrary, it is better to be as sensitive as possible in life. The skill of being accurately in touch with our feelings enables us to be more aware of what is really happening in the world (reality). We need to cultivate the feeling of what it would be like when things are going the way we would like. This creates the space which allows us to work, and attracts other possibilities.

When creating our lives we evaluate and construct our behaviour in terms of goals. The question we are asking is, what behaviour is required to accomplish what goals in the real world? The real world means right here right now. In the next moment or two reality may change drastically. Therefore what needs to be accomplished may dramatically change. Said differently, there is only the impermanence of each moment. For example we might be driving home from work planning an enjoyable dinner with our family. An automobile accident sends us to the hospital in critical condition. The planning and action change dramatically from one of creating a family dinner to one of what needs to be done to survive and recover. Reality has changed in a moment so our task is to change with it and re-evaluate what needs to be done.

This is what creating our life is. Seeing the impermanence and changeability of each moment, we act on the need of the moment. We simply do this continually until death. Nevertheless we need to create larger, long-term goals on which to base the structure of our moment-to-moment life. Then when we have to deviate from the activities of daily living we are more in tune with doing so. Each of us requires a list of priorities in life, or an understanding of what is important for ourselves. Otherwise there is no life to create. We just wallow in whatever is happening that moment and how we feel about it.

On six pieces of paper put the heading Priorities. On each piece of paper put one of the following subheadings:

• Lifelong • Mid length (5 -10 years) • Yearly • Monthly • Weekly • Daily

Our task is to list our priorities under each heading as life is viewed from this moment. The lists may be seen differently next week, next year or ten years from now. When we are creating life, these priorities will be in constant flux because a new moment brings unexpected demands and ways of seeing situations. Every moment we are a different person. We must regularly review and update our lists. This exercise may seem overwhelming but is a cornerstone in taking charge of a meaningful life.

Be as specific as possible. For example under Lifelong don't say to help others. What do we mean by helping others? Often by helping others in the short term we are disabling them in the long term. Why do you want to help others? There are many ways of helping others. If you truly mean it then give very specific examples of what action will take place. If you said to have a long happy family life, include specific descriptions of what your family life will look like and what actions will get you there. It is imperative you ask why you are making each choice. When you really understand why you made a particular choice you often realize that wasn't what you wanted after all. Try to list them in order of importance with the most important at the top.

Examples of Mid length priorities might be to complete my education (be specific), start a career (when, what career, doing what, where?), start a family (when, how do we financially support a family, who is the main caregiver?), down size my business (to what size, do I have the financial income to cope, what do I do with my time?) and so on. Be specific as possible.

Example of yearly goals might be to paint the house (who will do it, when, what colours?) lose weight (how, when do I start, what support do I have?), learn to play a musical instrument (what instrument, have I bought one yet, who is the instructor, can I afford it, when do I start?). Make your list as complete and specific as possible.

Likewise work on your monthly and weekly lists. You may notice they tend to revolve more around your job and family life. List deadlines and projects at work, personal and family commitments. List the family day at the zoo next Saturday. You must decide how high it goes on your list. Is it more important than repairing the lawn mower next Saturday? The more you struggle with this exercise the greater understanding you will have of what it means to create your life and see what is really important to you. The fact that you must act on your choices solidifies the process. You will be less thrown off by emergencies and general interruptions which must be attended to. You simply return to your list when you have dealt with these other issues, or new circumstances tell you to rewrite the list.

A daily list is extremely helpful in getting through the day in an expedient, productive way. Every evening sit down and create a priority list for the next day. On this list it is even more imperative to rank in importance the tasks of the day. At the top list the things that must be done. Realize it also includes personal time for yourself. If taking a walk tomorrow is important for you than it goes near the top and gets done. List all the tasks you want to complete tomorrow even if you know you can't accomplish them all.

Tomorrow start at the top of the list and work through the tasks. Since they are prioritized the most important ones get done. There may be a number of items left undone at the end of the day. That is fine. They may not have been that important so don't need to be done anyway. Or they may be put on a list for another day. As time passes it will become clearer to you that life is actually lived today, moment-to-moment, task-after-task. It puts a different perspective on wishing and hoping for something tomorrow. Things seem less urgent or less important.

Understanding that life changes each moment, be prepared to throw away the list for the day before even starting. You may receive an emergency phone call early in the morning that sets you on a different path for the day. That's fine, you are living a reality based life that must be attended to. Tomorrow will have its own list. Notice that all lists are based on looking at what is important for you, prioritizing, and acting on reality this moment. It becomes easier to accept the things you cannot change when you come to a deeper understanding that you have taken all the control you can and done your best.

A creative, purpose or goal orchestrated life will pay benefits of reduced anxiety and self-questioning. It will not eliminate our discomfort. Why should it? Anxiety, depression, sorrow and doubt are part of our interaction with life (reality). They are the barometer or measuring stick reminding us we are human beings experiencing life. Nevertheless we are still in charge of all our actions.

When in difficult or anxious moments we can ask ourselves several questions that will help:

- what is the real immediate problem?

- what is the source of the problem?

- what are the possible solutions?

- which solution can best be used?

The more often we use this approach the more we see there might not really be a problem. As we question the source we often see it is entangled in our attitude, perspective, emotions, beliefs and so on. A slight change of perspective on the situation often eliminates perceived problems.

In fact how can there be any problem in life? We know life is what it is, and we can't change that. We change our belief, cultural view, interpretation and we create our life through action based on reality. The choices of how to act in a given situation are not a problem because there are a limited number of choices. They are at worst a dilemma, as in which choice to make? For example say we equally enjoy chocolate and vanilla ice cream and are choosing one for dessert. This is not a problem. Reality has set the stage for us by saying we enjoy both flavours, those are the two flavours available, and it is prudent to have just one dish of ice cream.

Clearly this is about making a choice and nothing else, which we call a dilemma. In making this subtle but powerful shift in our view of life we are empowered to see all situations as a matter of choice. This will occur either beforehand by prioritizing and acting, or at the moment a more difficult decision must be made. We escape the tendency to dis-empower ourselves or remain stuck in an un-solvable situation by using the word *problem*. At worst we now see any situation as a *dilemma*.

Since life comes down to the choices of a dilemma our task is to determine which choice is warranted in a given situation. We need to be aware of emotional and cognitive responses. It is helpful to list two columns on a piece of paper, pros and cons, and fill in the columns as completely as possible. Sometimes it is best to wait a day or two before making a decision. We may add to the list in the meantime or interpret something differently. It is important to know our deadline and adhere to it. Making a decision by the deadline is empowering by itself. Remember, the decision is not necessarily about feelings, desires, likes and dislikes. What choice is needed?

We have created our priorities, created to-do lists and are living in the action of our lives. Great! We all know that demands are still placed upon us either gradually or acutely that infringe upon our priorities. These demands come from all sources but seem to emanate from work and family most often. An example may be the boss asking us to stay late tonight to complete a project. But we have committed seeing our son's soccer game. We need to clearly communicate to the boss what our priorities and commitments are, and negotiate an alternative proposal. Possibly coming in early in the next morning will be fine.

This is an example of *healthy boundaries* we have created in our lives. These might be described as the act of living our priorities and to-do lists within a healthy sense of reality. It is a boundary that protects us and others. Often it is not easy to negotiate a demand placed upon us. We must be firm and consistent on a regular basis. The more we behave in a firm consistent manner the easier it becomes. We are sending a message to the people around us. They learn the location of our boundaries, and are less apt to attempt to cross them when they realize they are firm. If a particular unhealthy situation is regularly repeated then further options might be explored. For example if the boss continually says no to negotiating alternative work times then maybe it is time to look for another position. This is in keeping with healthy boundaries and being in action.

Some people find it very difficult to create consistent boundaries. The need to sabotage our progress, or low self-esteem may be involved. It might be wise to seek feedback from others if we have difficulty creating healthy boundaries.

David Reynolds in his book *Water Bears No Scars* states, "We create stability and order through purposeful behaviour ... the order and stability exist as we create them by our doing ... what we are doing now isn't preparing us for self-improvement in the future. It either is self-improvement or it is not."

# Chapter 11
# *Living With Reality*

We understand clearly that no matter what the circumstances, we must change now - whether beliefs, attitude, awareness or actions. This is all we have to work with. What we do now creates who we will become tomorrow and in doing so changes the landscape of our circumstances. Stated differently, being with our discomfort of reality we must take charge right now. Dr. Shoma Morita a renowned psychiatrist, said, "self-development or changing doesn't aim to make life easy. It aims at making efforts to succeed even when we are failing." Therein lies our freedom.

The way we create identity or see ourselves is by how we see our past. So to change who we are is to change our past. We are creating a new past right now. What we do tomorrow will be part of our past. The more we are engaging we in the appropriate action of this moment the more different from before our past becomes. Each moment then empowers us to act in a more whole and confident way and to better deal with future dilemmas.

Living with reality today does not negate the fact that we live from a deeper Inner Life that is the core of our existence or primary purpose. The Inner Life is the Outer Life, or how we act now. The situation of the prisoners of war is a good example. Their Outer Life was whatever small things they could do to endure the hardships and survive. Their Inner Life was what drove them, what life was really about for each person. Life becomes simple flow the more we are in touch with our Inner Life. In other words the outward circumstances matter little as to what we need to endure. In fact the meaning of our Inner Life will tell us what needs doing no matter how difficult, and what is left is not really enduring but dealing with the way it is or our Outer Life.

Many of us wait until a crisis or extreme stress to ask what is our Inner Life? This opportunity can emerge at any point in our life and under any circumstances. But the chances are less that we can ask and receive an answer in a moment. If we are closing an important business deal, or looking after our family, we may want to call these tasks the meaning of our life. In a way they are. Whether the deal gets closed or not, what happens next? What happens when the kids grow up and don't need us? Obviously in some way the business deal and looking after our family are worthwhile endeavours. Meaning comes from a deeper position of timelessness and awareness. This is where our discussion of awareness from Chapter 5 comes in. Through deeper awareness we continue to reshape our Inner Life or meaning. We need to continually recognize when we are merely thinking about things instead of being aware. Obviously there is a place to think about things in particular circumstances.

This brings us back to completing the tasks of reality today. When we work with our Inner Life or meaning we are still left with what needs done here. There is no escape. Its just that the Inner Life has reaffirmed there is no alternative to what needs done now. We simply do it with more attention and simplicity, knowing we can't change the results. In a sense the actions of now become our power.

We are confronted with the question of success while living with the reality of today. Remember the prisoners of war. What was success for them each moment? Many of us have created tasks for today that we might consider in the success/failure conundrum. For example business deals, family tasks, promotions and so on. These issues create great stress when associated with desired outcomes. When we return to the notion that doing is infused with our Inner Life, then doing the simplest task right now is success. Now everything is complete. There is no stress!

## Characteristics of Living in Reality

- actions become habits that we call upon in stressful times

- worrying about the future is natural but useless

- it is natural but useless to be anxious in unknown situations

- we can only do one thing each moment

- complaining interferes with appropriate action

- creating small steps and goals is very productive

- the end result is in doing what needs done right now

- when we take care of our life, feelings take care of themselves

- events happen moment-to-moment, we don't create stories or tragedies out of them

- we accept our concerns and feelings and get on with cooking dinner

- fairness does not exist, life is simply event after event

- most people we consider great have suffered immensely

- live authentically and don't try to cure ourselves of anything

- we build character through seeing what needs done and then acting

- we face fear and do what we fear when appropriate

- we create and live with an internal feeling that everything is OK, even if things are not the way we want it to be

- we live life knowing no one is coming to rescue us, we are alone

- we take joy and meaning from the smallest of tasks

- we don't need immediate answers, just wonder

- we don't compare ourselves or our situation to another person's

- we are genuinely interested in others

- the world continues to look different as we change

- we engage in many passions and hobbies

- having a goal, means a having realistic means of achieving that goal

- we don't put our life on hold because of a dilemma, other things need to be done, and there is enjoyment to be had

- we keep doing

- we avoid, "I wish" or "if only" statements

- physical activity positively affects our emotions, so we are active

- there is always enough time; we create it

- we return everything we borrow

• we stop blaming others

• we admit when we make a mistake

• we keep our mental and physical lives in order

• we listen more and talk less

• we re-evaluate what success is

David Reynolds in his book *Constructive Living* states, "Each of us learns about Reality by living in it. Each moment of life is our teacher."

# Chapter 12
# *Self-Esteem*

Healthy self-esteem is essential in living a constructive, joyous life. It appears on a spectrum with none or a little amount at one end and abundant healthy amounts at the other. Most of us know our own feeling of personally being worthy, within a specific range on the spectrum.

Generally the higher our self-esteem the more we are engaged in life. We persist at tasks longer in order to meet what needs to be done. We have a sense of what is important to us, and have the efficacy to bring about the life we deserve. Through our life experiences each of us has a general sense of what level of self-esteem we embody. We have a clear understanding of how our life is orchestrated via our self-esteem. In other words, we are living the life we deserve. With low self-esteem our resilience to face challenging tasks is decreased.

In his book *Six Pillars of Self-Esteem,* Nathaniel Brandon defines self-esteem as, " the disposition to experience oneself as competent to cope with the basic challenges of life and as worthy of happiness." If we are going to construct a healthy lifestyle and be resilient to eventful situations we need an optimum level of self-esteem. Healthy self-esteem sets very specific expectations regarding what is possible in our reality. The actions we bring about deal with reality and in turn reinforce our level of self-esteem. The process continues. We are then more open to the realities of coping with the future. We can deal with life no matter what!

Resilience as discussed earlier has a great deal to do with this.

It is not the intent of the author to present a discourse on the topic of self-esteem. It is pertinent to raise the awareness of this critical topic. If the reader feels they personally need to work on this issue it is highly recommended they do so in whatever way is appropriate. It is pertinent to understand that the more choices and decisions we need to make at a conscious level, the more imperative our need for self-esteem.

Nathaniel Branden suggests people with healthy self-esteem carefully participate in weighing the following choices.

• focusing vs non-focusing

• thinking vs non-thinking

• awareness vs non-awareness

• clarity vs vagueness

• respect for reality vs avoidance

• respect for facts vs indifference to facts

• respect for truth vs rejection of truth

• perseverance vs abandonment of effort

• integrity in action vs disloyalty

• self-confrontation vs self-avoidance

• willingness to see and correct errors vs perseverance of errors

- reason vs irrationality

- loyalty to consciousness vs betrayal of the responsibility

Nathanial Brandon creates a list of some of the ways in which self-esteem manifests itself in us.

- self-esteem expresses itself in a face, manner, and way of talking and moving that projects the pleasure in being alive

- it expresses itself in an ease in talking of accomplishments or shortcomings with honesty

- it expresses itself in the comfort one experiences in giving and receiving compliments

- it expresses itself in an openness to criticism and a comfort about acknowledging mistakes

- it expresses itself in the harmony between what one says and does and how one looks, sounds and moves

- it expresses itself in an attitude of openness to and curiosity about new possibilities of life

- it expresses itself in the fact that feelings of anxiety or insecurity are not likely to intimidate or overwhelm

- it expresses itself in an ability to enjoy the humorous aspects of life

- it expresses itself in one's flexibility

- it expresses itself in one's comfort with assertive behaviour

- it expresses itself in relaxed, alert posture

Our self-esteem is affected by the choices we make each moment. What determines our level of self-esteem is what each of us does, within the context of our knowledge and values. This action is a reflection of action within the mind of the individual. Thus this process is an internal one.

Quoting Nathanial Brandon, "self-esteem is a consequence, a product of internally generated practices. We cannot work on self-esteem directly, neither our own or anyone else's."

There is much that might be said about self-esteem but the author is completely aware that if an individual recognizes a need, and is willing to address the issue he or she will create the resources to do so. We cannot live appropriately without the notion that we deserve life and are totally responsible for our actions. Self-esteem is critical.

# Chapter 13
# *Fear*

Our sense of fear is illusive and ever present. We all have fear, to a great extent buried in our consciousness where we aren't aware. It is one of the most powerful driving forces of our lives. It makes sense physically to protect oneself. When we are being chased by a grizzly bear we experience fear and realize it is prudent to get away. As an aside we may argue this is not fear but simply a prudent choice based on awareness, but that is another discussion.

How can we live responsibly when the impetus of our actions is greatly generated from a source we are not even aware of? We are continually living from a position of protecting ourselves emotionally. We are desperately attempting to protect our self-image, the story we have created about ourselves and life. It is impossible to live directly with the realities of each moment when we are instead living in this defensive illusion.

Let's return to the prisoners of war. There is the fear of being killed in the gas chamber, dying of starvation, being painfully beaten, and so on. We seem to create a mechanism or way of being that creates emotional walls around us. We become extremely afraid of being physically hurt. There is nothing wrong with this in some sense. Who would want to face this if they have a choice? But the very act of being afraid often prevents us from facing the truth of what has to be done this moment. It is more helpful to clearly see the grave situation and do what can be done, even if it is very little as in the case of the prisoners of war.

As Victor Frankl suggested it was when he confronted his fear of dying and saw it as the most likely thing to happen, he really could refocus and enjoy what he had. Minimal amounts of bread and soup sustained him, and even at that he gave much away to the other prisoners whom saw as weaker than himself. It was then he created better coping mechanisms and saw the the possibilities of escape (which never happened). The point is when we actually confront our fear and deal with reality the only way we can, that is as good as it gets.

Most of the prisoners had a self-image possibly of being middle class, business persons, family members, and so on. The experiences of the camp were most likely not congruent with their images or experience of life. Notions of, "its not fair, I can't survive, its too cold, too brutal" and more  probably orchestrated their lives. They built emotional walls to protect or maintain the image of what life should be like. This was fear. Again this prevented them from accepting what life really was for them. Therefore they couldn't adequately deal with the situation. Fear is the impetus to protect our self image, our view that life is to be a certain way. The result is stress. When we are aware of how fear operates then we are well on our way to observe our inappropriate actions.

Each of us might reflect on what self-images we are attempting to hold on to. We may want to maintain the image of a successful middle class person with an important job. We imagine this makes us look successful to others. We desperately try to maintain any image, resulting in great stress in our work place, family life and financial matters. Related to protecting our self image is the fact we are constantly comparing ourselves to others. Comparison is one of the greatest causes of fear, which becomes chronic stress. This leaves little energy or time to simply live life now.

We have an endless list of fears which propel our lives:

the fear of not being good enough, the fear of losing what we have, the fear of never having enough, the fear of being perceived as different, the fear of having less than others and so on. One of our major sources of chronic fear is the fear of looking at ourselves - the narcissistic, petty, superficial lives we live. Our fears show up in many ways in our daily life. It is the astute person who carefully observes their fears and takes appropriate action.

It is interesting to observe that fear is always in relation to something. It does not exist in an isolated state. For example we say we are afraid of not passing an exam or not being hired for a job. These fears are in a context. Our task is to deal with the question of being prepared for the exam, and looking at all the consequences of passing or not passing the exam. Then how can there really be fear?

To a great extent our fear is based upon the past or future. When we are prepared for an exam and have looked at the consequences of passing or not passing, and are still afraid, we are bringing the fear from the past and placing it upon the present situation. It is not fear resulting from the exam. Over time we have accumulated fear in not dealing with each situation realistically. Through habitual behaviour we constantly apply the fear from the past to now. It just seems like fear of the moment. Each day we feel anxious, and stressed.

A similar situation applies to the future. We have been so busy attempting to avoid realities of life it has become habitual. The anxiety becomes the state of the present moment. We are anxious about what happens next and how to avoid it. It is extremely helpful to understand where our fear is really coming from. When we are completely aware of the effects of fear now, we take appropriate action when dealing with matters only in the present.

Put another way, we like things to be a certain way. This gives us the feeling of security. We know things will be the same tomorrow, thus more security. If things are different tomorrow we move to a position of uncertainty or the unknown. There is a feeling of dissonance or stress. This ranges from how we store the coffee mugs on the shelf to the larger issues of life such as having a job, looking after the children, dealing with illness, death, and so on. We need to be aware of our nature to want life to be the way we usually know it. We are then more prepared to accept unknown situations and deal with them as best we can.

When we notice that we are constantly attracted to superficial pleasures, we can be confident that those behaviours cover vast fear that we are not in touch with. Obviously the term superficial pleasures is open to interpretation. Generally stated, they might be considered activities that do not bring deep, simple joy. They may not be within healthy personal boundaries. They don't seem to be connected to our responsibilities as stewards of this earth and its inhabitants. Observing this in ourselves is a significant step in understanding how our lives are driven by fear.

Jiddu Krishnamurti stated, "So there is in our life this constant state of comparison, competition, and the everlasting struggle to be somebody - or to be nobody, which is the same thing. This, I feel, is the root of all fear."

It is not reasonable to expect to be free of all fear. What is important is to recognize it, be in direct contact with it, understand where it is coming from, and get on with what needs to be done in the present.

# Chapter 14

## *Money*

Money has been elevated to a level of critical importance by so many of us. We probably are not aware of how we are driven by the pursuit of money. We justify it to ourselves by saying things such as we require it for the cost of food, housing, clothing, cars, vacations, children's education, electronic gadgets, and more. Yes these items do cost significant amounts of money. There is nothing wrong with money and the things it can purchase. In fact we can live very comfortably, enjoy ourselves and travel the world if we have enough money. In some respects it can't get any better. But we need to see money as a simple tool, and no more. Also, are we aware how we use it as a tool for comparing ourselves to another?

Money is a means to an end. If we have enough we can live any lifestyle we choose. That is wonderful! But money could not help the prisoners in the war camp. Money can not help us when we are ill (unless it pays for treatment). It probably has little use in watching a sunset or playing with a child. It can't help us when we are dead. Yes, we are going to die. Everything as we know it will be over. It can't help us in a moment of panic and stress. When we attend to this question of how money is meaningless to us the list becomes longer. It is a worthwhile exercise for the reader to explore the ways money has little value in his or her life. A more balanced overview of money may emerge. More options become available to us.

We can choose to move to a less expensive house or city. We may then change to a job making less money. The new job may be more fulfilling and less stressful. There are choices such as whether we own a car or rely on other forms of transportation. We can choose to spend less money on our lifestyle. In other words we can consciously choose any lifestyle we want, and it can be one with much less dependence upon money. Notice how difficult it is to contemplate this issue. We immediately want to compare ourselves to others and what they have or will think.

Often money is a vehicle by which fear operates. We all have been raised with particular attitudes about money. If messages were given that money is important, scarce, hard to come by, a status symbol and so on then we carry those attitudes today. Even if we have plenty of money we are still driven by our attitudes while growing up. We are still striving to earn more and not living the optimum life we might. Money in itself is neither good nor bad. We need to be clear on why we are working for it and how much we need and want. We need to understand where the impetus is coming from. On one hand there is a price to pay for earning money, but on the other hand it affords us wonderful things and opportunities. Look for many other wonderful activities to choose in life besides working for money.

In the end we are left with the realities we have. We need to do what needs done to pay the bills. Life is asking that of us. Our task is to do so with gratitude and enjoyment.

# Chapter 15
## *Relationship*

In our moment-to-moment daily life we are busy, striving to meet our needs and goals as we see them. It appears each of us is separate, in competition with the next person, grasping for whatever we can to survive or get ahead. Get ahead of whom or what? It seems few of us have really addressed this issue.

We have created the illusion each of us is separate here on earth, striving for our own individual purposes. Of course we are separate on a physical level. Each of us has our own aptitudes, strengths, weaknesses, passions and interests. But through our relentless striving we have developed a personal and cultural attitude of "me versus others."

As we observe nature we see that nothing exists in isolation. Trees are home and resting places for birds. Insects live in the trees. Trees give us shade and oxygen. Each animal has its particular position in the food chain. Plants are part of the food chain. Snow falls because of specific events in the atmosphere. The snow on the ground has an effect on the animals and plants. Storms come and go altering living circumstances for all of us. We could continue indefinitely reflecting on the intimate relationship between all things.

We are simply another species in the tapestry of all things. It is obvious each of us is not separate from anyone or anything else. We are affected by the movement of everything, and we affect everything else by our presence. No one or nothing escapes. From one point of view we might suggest we have little control as we are part of all things continually happening. Our lives are what is constantly happening. It becomes ludicrous to view life with the notion, "it should be this way or that." So when we are in touch with the natural relationship of all things we can't be surprised by events, anything happens any time. We are simply relationship with movement.

If we are bothered by people lying and the difficulties it creates we have several choices. We can view this as a personal attack on us, be stressed out and let others continue their lying. Or we can see it as an event with the movement of all events or things. Most would agree the world would be a better place if we were not lying. So understanding the relationship of all things and understanding our behaviour affects all else, we make the decision to be consciously aware of any small lies we might tell. We live our lives "squeaky clean" in other words. The impact on others is enormous. The people we affect in turn affect others. We have empowered ourselves and others by changing the initial stressor.

This opens the door to conscious choice of behaviour. Each choice allows us to stay up to date with the status of the moment. Decisions we made yesterday don't necessarily hold true today because everything (including us and our circumstances) continually changes. This is what is empowering for us. By keeping our choices "updated" we are always dealing with right now. This is living in the movement of relationship. Now we have control of our lives.

This turns our attention to responsibility. We cannot have relationship without responsibility, they go together. So no matter what happens, we have responsibilities. A major shift takes place. Our stress management strategies now incorporate the notion that we are responsible for ourselves and others, or all things. Of course this implies within a healthy reality and boundaries.

This is a shift away from self-centredness. Feelings of

isolation and separateness diminish. We feel more content. At more subtle levels we become aware of how we are affected by the actions of others and how we affect others. The more subtle our levels of awareness of interdependency become the more we want to change. Striving and stress are dramatically reduced.

Spend time reflecting on the relationship of all things, and the accompanying responsibility. We are a wave in the ocean.

# Chapter 16
# Simplicity and Balance

Our task is to live our lives simply. This means *deliberately choosing* each moment. We choose our life instead of being driven automatically. We are very clear why we make each choice. This means we are living consciously. Henry David Thoreau declared, "I went to the woods because I wished to live deliberately, to front only the essential facts of life, and see if I could not learn what it had to teach, and not, when I came to die, discover that I had not lived. I wanted to live deep and suck all the marrow of life ...." He did live austerely alone in the woods and face the essentials of life.

It was a remarkable awakening for Thoreau. The author does not suggest we all need to move to a log cabin in the woods, although it may be a wonderful experience. Simple, deliberate conscious living does not necessarily mean giving up our job, expensive car, large house, expensive restaurants and so on. On the other hand for some of us it may include doing those things. Ultimately it means making thoughtful, deliberate choices about each action while being aware of the consequences for ourselves and others. We then face the bare essentials of life. It is about the inner decisions we make. It is living from our essence as a human being. Jiddu Krishnamurti stated, "simple life does not consist in the mere possession of a few things." So don't give away the jewels and expensive car thinking things will change. We need to do more than that.

This essence can only unfold as we slow down, observe and deliberately act. We need to ask ourselves, "is this worth it, what am I really doing?" We need to give ourselves the space to find out, and then act. A basic level of needs and comfort are necessary for all of us. Unfortunately most of us choose not to stop. We experience a particular level of comfort and become addicted to it. We want more and more of the addiction. We lose sight of the fact that all we possibly need is food, shelter and clothing. So the issue is not whether we have wealth and possessions, or live a simple austere life, it is about the inner life we live in either case. Ralph Waldo Emerson reflected, "At night I went out into the dark and saw a glimmering star and heard a frog and nature seemed to say, well do not these suffice?"

Many of us claim we would live a different life if we had more time. At this moment we are alive so we do have the eternity of being alive, and chronological time. One hour from now we will do this or that. Also, any moment we will be dead, even thirty or forty years from now is any moment in the evolution of the universe. Reality is each breath, and is the only one we have because who knows what comes with the next one. After death we won't have any time, and it is coming quickly upon each of us. Life is precarious as time seems to be forever when alive, so we have enough and yet we don't have enough, and in the end it does not exist. Henry David Thoreau asked, "It is not enough if you are busy. The question is, what are you busy about?"

Time scarcity is something each of us creates. When we are constantly busy we do not have to face ourselves or others. We don't have to get to know anyone, especially ourselves. On the surface it looks like we give meaning to our lives when we are busy. We have accomplished this and that. This behaviour becomes very addictive. When we have a small open window of open time it is an uncomfortable situation and we quickly fill it. For the most part these are time fillers that separate us from living.

The way out of the dilemma is to look deeply at the time scarcity we have created. We must ask, "why, what am I escaping from, what am I going to do about this?" It is much easier to complain about the situation than take action. If we don't make the necessary changes, than it is obvious that we really don't want to, and the case is closed. When we have intention and commitment we find a way.

When we create space in our lives and slow down we notice the little things. There is so much to notice in the people around us. We see things in nature we never knew existed. We create loving kindness everywhere when the window of abundant time is open. We feel emotions that possibly we have have never really felt before. Approach time as something each of us own - something very sacred. Imagine your most sacred material possession. Now see your time as far more sacred than what you just imagined. It is yours until death, nurture it and keep it your own. It will provide you with vastly more than you could ever dream possible.

This raises the issue of time boundaries. Like anything in life, if we don't nurture and protect it, it will be gone. Those around us have ways of stealing our time. Or putting it another way, they cunningly convince us to give it away. We give it away because we want their approval. Why? Who are they? We need clear predetermined boundaries in place before the demands begin. We need to be aware of how guilt and threats will be used against us. The response is simple, **No**. When we have difficulty saying this we need to look at underlying issues such as self-esteem, need to placate and so on. The majority of people tell us they have more respect for those who know their needs and wants, and will stand up for them. Mohandas Gandhi said it as well as anyone, "A *no* uttered from the deepest conviction is better than a *yes* merely uttered to please, or worse, to avoid trouble."

Sue Bender writes in her book *Everyday Sacred*, "I wanted to see everyday life with fresh eyes. What might have been there all along that I had not been able to see? What had I taken for granted?" This is living, the real thing! We need to streamline our lives to have time for the things that matter. We need to ask ourselves whether what we are doing this moment will contribute to what is important in our lives. If not, why are we doing it? Thich Nhat Hanh wrote, " Every morning we have twenty-four brand new hours to live." What does the reader plan on doing about the next twenty-four hours?

"The essence of simplicity is living from the core of our being," as stated by Janet Luhrs in her book *The Simple Living Guide.* This applies to living in a concentration camp, coping with a narcissistic boss, or looking after an ill child. In all cases what needs to be done comes from the same inner core of who we are. Our core being does not change, only our outer circumstances. We no longer have to look for answers outside ourselves, so we don't complicate our lives. Life is what we choose it to be this moment. Aldous Huxley in his book *The Perennial Philosophy* stated, "a person's single most important task is to discover the divinity of ordinary things, ordinary lives, and ordinary minds." The importance of this statement can not be overestimated. Stop running on automatic pilot. Look!

Living simply is often equated with doing or having less. This is a common desire among those with complicated, seemingly out-of-control lives. Yet this is a dangerous supposition as suggested earlier. As we simplify, we discover that we don't necessarily want to do less or have less. Rather we want to consciously choose what we do, instead of feeling endless obligations from external forces. Living simply gives us this freedom. It is critical to see this.

One possible simple model for living a balanced life is to imagine a square and visualizing the four corners being four pillars of our lives. Our lives are then lived within the sides of the square. The four pillars are myself, family, job and community.

The first pillar is myself. We must have a healthy sense of

ourselves, meaning a sense that we deserve the best in life, are willing to reach for it, and have many interests, hobbies and passions. It includes looking after our own mental and physical health. We are engaged in life. We are responsible to see to it that all these things happen. If we are not as complete and responsible a person as possible than we are not bringing assets to our families, job and community. Each must take time to create an appropriate personal life that is structured around his or her own healthy needs and wants.

Outside of our personal life, the cornerstone is family life. Family life is an important cornerstone of our society. Everyone has the responsibility to explore what family life means to themselves and other family members. If we recognize we are not spending appropriate amounts of time engaged in family activities we seriously need to inquire why not?

We do not live an isolated existence. We are part of numerous communities that might be represented by concentric expanding circles moving from a centre. We are part of the community of the street we live on. We have a responsibility to participate in the activities that shape life on our street. Similarly we are part of a town, city, country and indeed everything that exists. Obviously we must select where and how we will contribute to our community. This is based upon our interests, strengths, weaknesses, time restraints and so on.

We have the most effect on our immediate surroundings and circumstances. It is suggested that is where most of our community time and energy be spent. That is not to say we should not get involved in an issue halfway around the world. There may be much to contribute. But we are responsible for life in our community here and now. The goodness of life in our community then spreads to other parts of the world. When we don't create an appropriate life in our space we can't expect to create significant changes anywhere else. Each of us needs to work out for ourselves what and how we have to contribute. Examples of community work may be: volunteer work at the hospital, Boy Scouts, coaching children's sports, serving on a community social committee, or replacing dying trees in town.

Most of us require a job for obvious financial reasons. The job will take significant amounts of our time and energy. It is wise to have a job we enjoy, and one that contributes appropriately to our community. Some who don't require a job for financial reasons still work for enjoyment and to contribute. Wonderful! As stated earlier, stress accumulates as we gradually realize we are spending inordinate time doing things in our lives that are not meaningful or supportive of our surroundings. It is better to always be vigilant and aware of what we are doing in our job, and be willing to make immediate changes.

When we see our lives can be balanced within these four pillars, our existence shifts. We are not merely trying to survive as an individual, but have intentionally committed to participate in four major areas of life. This creates the sense of control. We have input into what is happening in our lives. We are not relegated to the position of victim of what is happening outside ourselves. We create what is happening, we *are* life. What joy!

# Chapter 17
## Order

Whether we are busily involved in many areas of life or have significant time on our hands, order is essential. Order is what needs to be done this moment to be efficiently open to the next moment and what its responsibilities bring. It is not doing any more than necessary, but doing what needs done. It is doing more than needs to be done without concern. It is having what is required. It is having beyond what is required. It is getting things done in the simplest, most efficient manner. It is a state of mind. Then the things that need done, get done.

When we are balancing our chequebook we have a few minutes or all day to complete the task. It does not matter. It means having the chequebook, a pen or pencil, all statements and records and whatever else is needed. These items are easily accessed because we know where they are kept. We have an uncluttered spot to sit and work. It is always available because we keep things that way. We work without interruption unless it is an emergency. We make that clear to all family members. We do only the task we set out to do. We do not answer the phone, begin cooking or anything else. When we are finished balancing the chequebook we return everything to where it is usually kept. We are prepared for the next time.

This lifestyle is essential whether we are busy or not. It is about orchestrating our lives to run smoothly. Even when we are not busy, without order we feel rushed, frantic and stressed. Order shows up in arranging our furniture in the simplest and tidiest possible way. Order is eliminating all the tools and gadgets we don't need. We can't find them any way, and they prevent us from finding other things we do need. Order is cleaning our house on a regular basis even if we don't think it is necessary. All of a sudden it is necessary, and we feel overwhelmed because the job is much harder now.

Order is about having less, but everything we need, without going to extremes. It is about having more than we need, without being attached to more and appreciating and enjoying the blessings. It is being comfortable. It is being uncomfortable without resistance. It is our mind being smooth and simple. It is the movement of all things. Each of us must find our own notion as how to be with this. It is a state of mind in which we see and are the organized flow of our lives. The actions automatically follow.

Remember, from past experience we all have created a map in our mind as to what life is supposed to be. The more the reality of this moment differs from our map, the more stress we sense. We feel anxious, depressed, angry, or irritable. We create stories about how we can't cope, saying this is awful, blaming someone, and so on. In other words it appears as chaos to us. Being the creatures we are, we like everything to make sense and want to be in control. So our task is to see our present situation as real (we don't have to like it), which it is, being aware of how we label it chaos, and understanding we change it by creating order in our perspective, thinking and actions. We make order out of chaos.

Whether we are trying to cope with living in a concentration camp, busily preparing for a dinner party or washing kitchen dishes our task is the same. Often we label it as chaotic because it doesn't fit our internal map. Therefore we need to reduce the situation into small, sequential, manageable pieces of what needs to be done. Now we are coping, getting by and in control. We recognize this as OK. We just notice all thoughts and feelings about the situation. So we get on with life, creating a predictable, manageable, tailor-made sense of what is happening. These actions change our feelings anyway. That is all we have to do. Its over! Order itself takes over and sees us through.

Getting things done is one of the most important skills we can master. This is order. It is not necessarily about things viewed as "work," such as completing a report or cutting the grass. It is also going for a walk, going to the movies, taking a bath or having a glass of wine. What is important?
What are the needs of the situation? Doing this is order.

Our struggles of what to do generally fall into one of two categories. We know what needs done, but choose not to do it. Secondly, we really don't know what to do. Most of the time, most of our lives are spent in the first scenario. There is little more that can be said. We can't expect to win the ball game when we don't show up to play. The second scenario may be viewed as more challenging.

Our usual behaviour of just "keeping busy" and hoping we cover all the bases is inappropriate. We already know our "busyness" is only to block ourselves from seeing ourselves, seeing the truth. When do we get to things that really need done? How do we know what really needs done? This is a challenging question? Each moment is fresh and new, even when we are doing nothing or bored. The complete universe changes each moment. Therefore each new moment brings another something-to-be-done, even if nothing. There is no alternative.

The issue of what needs done is often presented to us in a disguised way. It appears complicated or opaque. Our task is to see through this. Unfortunately we distract ourselves by thinking about ourselves, our situation, ruminating over feelings, applying our philosophy, or focusing on one small aspect of the situation. In other words, **we** are the problem, as we usually are. We need to let our natural mind be open and flexible to the ever changing moment. In a sense, life tells us what to do, and there is no alternative.

We need to spend our energy being aware of our own impediments suggested in the above paragraph. Just being aware of their presence is the greatest step in seeing beyond them. Now we are simply left with paying attention. For example, we see the garden needs attended to. Then it gets attended to now. Our impediments that stopped us before are now gone. There is no alternative but attend to the garden now. If we are leaving for work when we observe the garden, we automatically perform the task at the first reasonable opportunity.

Paying attention tells us that numerous things need done. We know that means now. Reality tells us we can't do more than one thing at a time. We have a dilemma. We can't do everything right now that we see needs done. We must prioritize. Now only one thing needs done. Everything is now complete.

To prioritize we need to reflect on some of the questions we have used before. What is the purpose of doing this, what will be the impact on myself and others, how urgent is this, how much does it fit into our greater purpose? The key is to step back and reflect. Create a pause in our momentum. Clarity is present. In the end, there is a flow or momentum that seems to be beyond us and yet is us, and our lives are lived with little effort. This is order.

# Chapter 18
# *Luck*

Everything Jane touches smells like a rose. My life would be so different if I had her luck. How often do we think or say this? Jane's life may look better than ours. We know that statement comes more from our perception, beliefs, interpretation and so on. Jane may see her own life very differently than we do and view her life as an ongoing struggle. What is really wrong with my life anyway, we might better ask?

So often we escape our responsibilities this moment by assuming peoples lives are orchestrated by good luck and ours just happens. We know this does not work and increases our distress. Yes, sometimes difficult situations arise and tragedies happen. Sometimes it appears they happen to us, and not to others. Some things work out, some don't. Someone wins the lottery, and someone does not. Is this luck? What is luck? Would our life really be different if our luck was different? Who knows, but that is most likely up to the individual involved.

There is significant room to suggest that we have considerable control over what happens to us, during what appear to be random events. This is about taking control of the things we can control. It is about creating our lives and increasing our self-efficacy instead of seeing ourselves as helpless or victims of life. We know that doing what needs to be done reduces our stress.

In his book *The Luck Factor,* psychologist Richard Wiseman

strongly suggests that there is a lot more to luck than mere chance. He states we can understand why many seemingly chance things happen, and we can actually influence them too. The key, he continues, is recognizing that pure chance is almost non-existent. After many years of research he has identified four characteristics that make some people luckier than others, or, by applying these behavioural principals we improve our own luck. In other words, we choose to make things happen in our lives.

We can choose to:

## 1. Make the most of random opportunities:

Let's view life as a spectrum with chance at one end and control at the other. For the most part, our lives take place somewhere in the middle. All we need to do is slide ourselves little by little toward control. The obvious way of changing how things happen is to seize every random opportunity, large or small, to change our luck. Lucky and unlucky people have the same number of random opportunities. The difference between the two is that the unlucky don't see and act on the opportunities. The lucky ones pay attention and see opportunities others don't. Acting on an opportunity may include uncomfortable situations like talking with strangers, or acting on an appropriate hunch.

Lucky people tend to be more relaxed, even in pressure situations, which affords them opportunities to spot lucky breaks. Lucky people vary their routine, do different things, drive on different roads and so on that allow new opportunities to rise.

## 2. Act on lucky hunches:

Whether we call it a hunch, gut feeling, intuition or our subconscious, this is how we make many daily decisions. We might walk away from someone because of the tone of his voice, while we strike a business deal with someone else who has a different tone. Yet we are not aware of why we acted the way we did. Gut level decisions aren't something we always recognize we are making, so when the results are positive, they feel more like random events than they are.

If something "seems or feels right," chances are it is. If something "seems  wrong or inappropriate," chances are it is. The more we act on hunches the better we become with this skill.

### 3. Expect good fortune:

A significant difference between a hockey player who scores 50 goals in a season and one who scores 10 goals is that the one who scores 50 goals expects to. This applies to all areas of life, business, love, sports and so on. At some level each of us has created an upper limit of success we will reach. For most of us, most of the time we have given up before we start. We receive what we ask for.

### 4. Turn bad luck into good:

People who have been through difficult times often demonstrate more resilience and persistence than the rest of us. They turn unfortunate circumstances into goodness. They realize that very often it is the only thing they can do. What appears to be good luck is really using a tapestry of inner strengths to create something new. Most of us have heard about turning lemons into lemonade.

## Chapter 19
# *Mistaken Identity*

We are not who we think we are. We have a self-image based upon how we have interpreted the events of our lives. We think our lives are created by events and we are afraid of losing control of ourselves, thus losing control of events, or having a fear they may happen again. Right now we are living the story of our self-image, not the reality of the moment. This is the story that tells us whether we can survive the next crisis, another day with the boss, the demands of children, or preparing for the dinner party. This is what creates our beliefs and limited awareness. When we believe we are not good at skiing ... well, we aren't. We live our lives each moment with the "shackles" of our identity orchestrating everything. This is the person we identify with.

But what if we are not this person? What if this story has been made up and we just memorized it to be our story? Then who are we? Do we notice more anxiety rising when we ask that question? What if we are not the anxious person who can't handle business meetings? It is easier to live with lies and self-deceit than face something we don't know. That is what we do.

Remember we have learned that the greater the dissonance between our story or map of life and the reality of this moment, the greater the stress we feel. Our story or map of life is really just our self-image. If we didn't have a particular self-image who is to say what we can and cannot handle? Stress only shows up when we fear we cannot keep reality in line with our story of who we are, and what we can handle. So if we change our story of who we are, life will be a lot different. It will be much simpler. We will successfully deal with each situation as it arises.

Why don't we change our self-image or story? The answer is we must give up our past. It has already gone, anyway. The real dilemma is the fear of giving up the past. If we give it up, the question then arises, "who am I?" The past has gone, we are really holding on to our feelings and thoughts from the past with the illusion that they will protect us from something happening again. That is what keeps us stuck right now. Otherwise we have no identity from the past. Our task then is confronting the fear of giving up the thoughts and feelings of the past, which in turn frees us to live openly right now, able to deal with anything. Then who will we be? Interesting ...

Even when we aren't knowingly identifying with the past but are scurrying, trying to get more done now, we are still driven by holding or reacting to the thoughts and feelings of the past. We cannot escape until we aware of what is going on. What we want to do is *feel* different, not be different. We feel different by letting go of our feelings about the past. Then we are different. Life will now unfold in a different manner because we are actually different.

The more we are thinking about or focusing on ourselves the more we are strengthening our limiting self-image. Said differently, the thoughts, feelings, ideas and so on that we ruminate over are our identity and restraining shackles. So instead of reflecting on these things, we need to just get on with life, doing what needs done this moment. The person we think we are is no longer there to make things difficult. Now things get done, events occur, we are content, and life flows on.

We break free of thoughts and feelings by seeing that even though it may feel that way at the moment, we are not owned by them. We are only temporarily occupied. Seeing this important distinction instantly changes our attitude toward any stressful situation that intimidates us into giving it authority over our lives.

Taking control and seeking power are two completely different issues. We seek power, overtly or covertly, because we are dominated by our feelings, whether we know it or not. We believe something outside ourselves is causing our unhappy or disturbing feelings. So we seek power over someone or something to solve the problem of wanting power over our feelings. It never works. The more stressful the situation the more we are tempted to seek power to solve it. No one seeks power to do good. Taking control is simply for the overall benefit of the situation. We need to be vigilant.

Stress exists because we insist. Our wish to have power over life comes from a wrong relationship with life. Reality has its own effortless course. We don't need power to flow.

# Chapter 20
# *Relaxation*

A basic fact of life is we all experience tension and anxiety as part of our existence. We emotionally and physically respond to the everyday stressors of life. Depending on temperament and circumstances the experiences can be mild or agonizingly severe. So most of us need to practice regular relaxation techniques to maintain optimum health.

*Anxiety* may be a word that is overused today and thus difficult to define. Nevertheless we might refer to it as the reaction we have to a situation where we believe our well-being is endangered or threatened in some way. When we say a person is nervous we may well be suggesting they are anxious. *Tension* may be thought of as chronic, usually low level anxiety that is experienced as part of an ongoing situation in which we are involved. *Fear* may be thought of as tense anxiety experienced in response to a specific threat. Anxiety in moderate amounts motivates us to plan for future events and increase our ability to cope with situations as they occur. It is when anxiety becomes excessive that it is a difficulty. It inhibits optimum performance.

Our objective is to keep the nervous, and voluntary and involuntary systems functioning at optimum level. For example our breathing is an involuntary action but under stress breathing becomes shallow and rapid. This physiological response reinforces the effects of the stressor. In this case our job is to reclaim normal deep relaxed breathing. With ongoing stress our muscles tighten. When stress is reduced usually our muscles relax. This is *acute stress* when the duration of stress is relatively short and the muscles relax after each episode. When the periods of stress become longer and more frequent then it is seen as *chronic stress*. The muscles have greater difficulty relaxing between episodes.

## Slow Deep Rhythmic Breathing

The most basic, and possibly the most important method of relaxing is practising deep, slow, rhythmic breathing. It slows down our quick shallow breathing resulting from stress, and has a direct impact on all our body systems. We slow down all bodily functions which allows the systems to relax and work efficiently. We are delivering more oxygen to every cell in the body. In a more efficient way we are removing waste products from each cell, as cells accumulate more waste products when under stress. The waste products themselves if left unchecked become an additional stressor. The reasons are numerous to view deep, slow breathing as a primary stress reducer.

This stress management technique requires no equipment, no financial expense and is completely portable. It can be practised anywhere or anytime. There are many views as to how it should be practised. It is the intent here to present a simple method of getting maximum benefit from the exercise. Each individual might consider exploring what is best for them. Ideally, situate yourself in a quiet, comfortable location and begin to notice your breathing. Are you breathing from the chest or abdomen? Slowly begin to breath deeper, extending the abdomen within a comfortable range. Allow the air to flow out without forcing. Develop a slow rhythmical cycle. Now just watch, be aware of your breathing. If you notice breathing becoming shallower or faster, gently make appropriate adjustments.

A comfortable time frame to practice might be twenty minutes. A benefit of this technique is that if you only have five minutes of time it is still very beneficial. Notice how the body relaxes, breathing slows down and deepens, and you feel more relaxed and calm. This technique can be used during a stressful business meeting. Sit back and refocus, begin using your deep breathing. No one else will notice and within several minutes you will be more relaxed, calm and recharged.

Create the habit of slow deep breathing in any situation. For example take several minutes when busily engaged with the children. It can be used during an anxiety provoking phone conversation. Better yet, develop the habit of practising it numerous times every day no matter where you are or what you are doing. Just sit back and begin. When practised numerous times each day the effects are cumulative and become preventive. You are more prepared for the stressful moments. Each breathing break is a mini vacation from what you are currently engaged in. The effect of a momentary break is in itself a stress reliever.

## Visualization

This technique also requires no equipment, no financial expense and is completely portable. We all have our favourite activities, or locations in the world. From experience, we know being there creates a peaceful, restful climate within ourselves.

During stressful situations sit back, check your breathing and visualize or picture yourself performing your favourite activity. It may be skiing down your favourite mountain in the Alps. Picture it clearly in your mind. Add as many details as you are familiar with. Feel being there with your whole body. You are completely removed from what you were just doing. Now use all your senses if possible. This adds realism. Feel the cold air on your face. Listen to the cutting edge of the skis in the snow. Notice the details of the trees. Smell the freshness of the air. Be there with your total being. You will notice when it is time to return to your activity of studying or the business meeting. You are more refreshed.

Most of us have a constellation of favourite activities or places that can be used for this activity. Create a list ahead of time so when required you already have a menu to draw from. Another favourite may be lying on the warm, soft sand of a tropical island. Be there by using detail, feel it, enjoy it. Like deep breathing you can use this technique every day as preventative medicine. Make a habit of using twenty minutes a day for this practice. The benefits are extraordinary.

## Progressive Muscle Relaxation

It is quite simple to train ourselves to relax our muscles. Relaxed muscles lead to a relaxed body and mind. This technique also does not require expensive equipment and is portable. When relaxation exercises are practised regularly, our levels of tension and anxiety can be reduced significantly. Just as physical exercise trains and strengthens our muscles, relaxation exercises increase our ability to tolerate stress and remain calm during moments of life's pressures.

Sit in a comfortable chair, lie on a couch or lie on the floor. Check your breathing, begin slow deep breathing. Tell yourself you are relaxed while you visualize being relaxed. Focus on the muscles of your head and scalp. Feel them. Tell yourself they are relaxing. Feel them relax. Allow each wrinkle in your forehead to smooth out. It is the natural flow of things, just let it happen. Take as much time as required. Check your breathing. Now move to your face. Say, I will relax the muscles of my face. Feel them, let them relax and go limp. We hold tension in our jaws. Let the jaw go. Spend as much time as required with the face. Next focus attention on the neck muscles. Let them become tranquil and allow the tension to drain away. Take the required time.

Slowly continue through the remainder of the body repeating similar exercises. Move to your shoulders, down your arms, through your wrists, hands and fingers. Return to your chest, letting go of all tightness. Keep checking your breathing. Move to your stomach muscles, then proceed to your back. Relax all muscles up and down your spine, waist, buttocks, thighs and hamstrings. Proceed down the calves, ankles, feet and toes. Continue to lie there and allow the body to go limp. Very slowly get up, check breathing, and integrate with the next activity.

After several sessions you will notice how relaxed you have become. Repeat this exercise on a daily basis. For some individuals it helps to purposely tense the muscles of that part of the body being worked on. Then immediately relax those muscles after the forced tension. This teaches us to discriminate clearly between a tense and relaxed state. For many of us our muscles are so chronically tight we are not even aware of it. This has become our natural state. A few daily exercises will work wonders.

Each of us has our own particular locations for storing muscular tension. The more we practise the exercises the more we learn where our individual "hot spots" are in the body. We can then choose to spend more time in our hot spots when doing the exercises. Examples of common hot spots are the neck, jaw and lower back. We need to tailor make this exercise to meet our individual needs. With practise we learn how best to spend time on the various muscle groups.

We can use a varied option of progressive muscle relaxation during any stressful moment of the day. When feeling tense during a business meeting, sit back and check your breathing. You can quickly scan the body from head to toe performing the exercises. Alternatively you can choose to zero in on your hot spots for several minutes. The effects will be felt very quickly.

## Systematic Desensitization

Many of the anxieties that we experience are due to what we call conditioned reactions. Things that frequently occur together in our experience become linked or associated with each other so that we respond to them in the same or similar way when they happen again. Thus if we are made anxious or afraid in the presence of certain factors (stimuli), these same factors will make us anxious later when they occur, even if the situation in reality no longer poses a threat.

For example, if someone had one or more experiences in the past where they felt they were endangered by raw food, their reaction today to raw food might produce more anxiety than the situation calls for. This may include the sight, smell or even thought of raw food. This is because of their previous conditioning of anxiety to this food. So this person may become anxious any time by the mere thought of raw food. Many of our emotions seemed to be largely dependent on such conditioned reflexes.

Such conditioned reflexes can be overcome through systematic desensitization. Each scenario is unique so a program must be tailor made. Generally, continuing our example, we expose ourselves to descriptions, pictures, or samples of the exact foods that we react to. This is done in a relatively safe and systematic way so that we are exposed to the least anxiety provoking stimuli first and the most anxiety provoking at the end.

Begin each session by completely relaxing using the techniques you know. Now look at the piece of food (photo, etc.) that stimulates the least anxiety. Close your eyes and imagine yourself present with this image. When anxiety rises switch to feeling totally relaxed using your relaxation techniques. Alternate back and forth from being with the food and images, to relaxing. By the end of the session you will feel much more comfortable. This session may be repeated numerous times before moving on to the next desensitization phase involving another food, or situation with food.

The more one practises this exercise the greater the desensitization. This method can be used with almost any conditioned reflexes such as fear of flying, insects or public speaking. In more complicated cases it may be helpful to seek support from someone trained and experienced with this technique.

## Meditation

The word meditation is a very overused word, that has evolved from people putting a "contemporary spin" on it, and creating a commercial enterprize. Each person has their own interpretation of what it means. There are numerous religious, spiritual and business organizations competing for the attention of the consumer. It is not the intent of the author to review or endorse any particular practice. This inquiry is the responsibility of the each individual to best determine what meets his or her own personal needs and tastes.

The significant point is to create personal quiet time each day for possibly twenty to thirty minutes to allow the mind to slow down and the body to relax. With the hustle of our daily activities our minds tend to race with ideas, problem solving and so on. Then we are not aware of what is really going on, thus not doing what needs to be done, if anything. We need to break this cycle.

Choose a quiet place, sit comfortably, loosen any tight clothing and close your eyes. Check your breathing and relax. Be aware of your breathing but do not try to change or control it. Sit and watch your breathing. Just sit, watch. Emotions and thoughts will enter the mind/body. Observe them, be with them, let them go when the time is appropriate. Return to observing the breath. Thoughts and feelings are simply a product of thousands of years of evolution of the mind/body. For the most part they have no significance, in fact they are often our downfall because we spend most of our lives reacting to them. We may notice that one or two appear to have particular significance regarding our lives. This might be noted and the thought or feeling be furthered explored, or in the future the thought or feeling can be further explored.

A daily practice of quiet time will significantly reduce stress and better enable one to cope on a daily basis. This technique is portable and can be used any time. One can use it on a subway, during a business meeting, or simply sitting at your desk.

## Biofeedback

Biofeedback might be seen as a constellation of methods giving us direct feedback as to how muscles, organs, or brain wave patterns are actually functioning. We then have the opportunity to explore ways of altering their functioning and changing our stress level. We learn more appropriate long term coping strategies.

Biofeedback usually involves technical equipment and direction from  trained personnel in the medical/counselling field. There are many types of programs and equipment available. It is suggested that one seriously explore all options before going ahead with this technique. Results can be very beneficial.

# Chapter 21
## *Vacations*

We have all met the person who says he has not missed a day of work in twenty years, and, even more impressive, never had a vacation. They claim to feel great and couldn't be happier. That may be true, but how does one know the mountain if he has never experienced the valley, or vice versa? When we live life on automatic we are not aware of anything else. The issue is we don't know we are living on automatic. Stated differently, we don't know what we don't know.

We can suggest numerous reasons for taking a vacation every year, whether one, two, three or more weeks. The emotional and physical effects of stress are cumulative. Often it is too late when we realize stress is building. We must live proactively, taking charge of our lives each moment. We need to be responsible for our health now.

If we suggest our purpose in life is to be happy, responsible participants in the world, then we need to step outside the framework of our job and participate in the world from a different viewpoint. When we do this we are removing ourselves from the daily routine, which in itself is often a shock because we are addicted to it. Even to wonder what else there is in life is a step forward. We are breaking the stress cycle. We are looking beyond ourselves, wondering, moving toward becoming a more complete person. The more eclectic and balanced our lives are the more relaxed we are. We are more engaged in life, and interesting to others.

The exciting news is that vacation does not necessarily mean an expensive trip to an exotic part of the world, which we probably can't afford anyway. Vacation may mean spending two weeks cleaning the garage, thus finding an old bicycle and baseball glove long forgotten. It means seeing and talking to the neighbours while cleaning the garage. It means working at your pace. It means accomplishing something that has needed done for years. What a great feeling! The point is to change physical location, engage in a different activity with different expectations, and receive no direction from others. It does not really matter what we do.

We may spend a vacation engaged in hobbies such as scuba diving, photography, cooking, gardening or reading. We may spend a vacation lying on the beach or hiking a remote mountain. It is about changing gears for a while. It is about passion. It is about taking complete responsibility for our lives, if only for a short period. Notice how many people you have known, who at the end of a vacation, have said they are not returning to their job. The small break was enough for them to realize there is more to life, and choose some other form of work. Often they walked away from large salaries and fancy titles on their door.

The notion of vacation is not viewed as only one break per year. Look at the cycle and stress of the other remaining weeks during the year. Let's view a vacation as any break, no matter what length, from the the routine of what we are doing. This now creates limitless possibilities! Taking vacations every month, every week, every day, and possibly viewing life as one long vacation. Yes, ultimately that's what life is, simply for the choosing.

Every weekend or other days off is viewed as a vacation. We have twenty-four or forty-eight hours to do what ever we choose. Once every one or two months, go away for a weekend. View it as a vacation. Go to a resort, take a hiking trip or simply follow your passion. Can't afford it? Every weekend is viewed as a vacation, even by staying home. Consciously choose to engage in activities that you are passionate about, and you are still removed from your job and other responsibilities. They may include taking walks, going to the movies, cooking gourmet meals and so on. The length of time spent on an activity is not as important as seeing it as vacation time. During one weekend we may participate in five or more different activities, or vacations. When was the last time you took five separate vacations during one weekend? Try it!

Our common reaction to this suggestion is we have to grocery shop, do laundry, etc. on the weekend. Remember, we are making a deliberate, conscious shift in our attitude and lifestyle. At first it takes effort. If we are serious about this we have already dealt with many of these chores during the week by rearranging our schedules to accommodate our vacation weekends. For any chores still left for the weekend, view them as vacations instead of chores. For example, if the grass needs mowed view it as a walk through a park, while physically and emotionally energizing yourself. This shift in consciousness has amazing affects. If we still have shopping to do, view it as a vacation or break from other aspects of the weekend. When we are alive, healthy and happy nothing feels like a chore, everything is a gift. Try it!

Each weekday we can add vacations as well. View the time period from waking to before leaving for work as an opportunity for multiple small, or mini vacations. Keep in mind we are not acting from the position of automatic responses, but conscious choices in which each activity is a break from the previous one and there is a moment of rejuvenation each time. We can review the newspaper without rushing, or trying to read it completely, but seeing it as a joyful activity in itself. We may look out the window for several minutes to observe the weather and the beauty of today. The shift is away from, do I need to wear a coat today, to seeing this as a precious, unique moment. What a pleasant surprise! Enjoy a few minutes of sitting, eating breakfast and actually tasting the food. If we don't eat breakfast before work, changes are required. Breakfast is the most important meal of the day. We require the nutrition to physically and emotionally function at optimum performance. Besides, breakfast is an enjoyable mini-vacation itself.

So, before leaving for work we can participate in as many mini-vacations as we choose, each one being different and enjoyable. But what if we don't have time? Remember, the answer is always the same; do what needs to be done this moment. Set the alarm clock for twenty minutes earlier.

Whether driving to work or going by bus we have more vacation time. Albeit we must be more aware and alert when we are driving. But the drive is a vacation from being at work, and from being at home having breakfast. It is an activity of its own. We just need to be present while driving and deal with what comes up each moment. Sitting on the bus is truly a magnificent vacation. We may practise any of our relaxation techniques, read, simply observe the surroundings or be in gratitude. All for the price of a bus ticket!

We may have busy pressure-filled days at work, but they can be spent with numerous mini-vacations. Sitting at our desk, or with any task, we can momentarily physically pull back from what we are doing, refocus, check our breathing, visualise being somewhere else or progressively relax some muscles. When returning to work within a minute or so we are energized, replenished and have a more realistic view of what we were doing. We have broken the "being on automatic" pattern. These mini- vacations may be taken dozens of times per day. We may suggest we are losing productive work time, but in reality we are much more productive during a day's work.

An exciting mini-vacation at work is a visit to the washroom. In the past we may have viewed this as an intrusive interruption from our work. But view it as a vacation, a trip or journey of its own. While walking to the washroom observe the surroundings, speak to people, listen to the noise, smell the air and feel the exercise. Look around the washroom like you never have looked before, as if it were an exotic island you have never visited. Observe the details of the washroom. You will be surprised! Don't think about what you have to do back at your desk, you are on vacation for several minutes. Upon returning take a different route, take note, smell, listen, and enjoy yourself.

Trips to the water fountain and coffee pot are also viewed as mini- vacations. Don't go for a drink of water while "on automatic." Anticipate the excitement and adventure of the walk and the drink of water. Observe the surroundings, listen, talk to people, feel your legs stretch and actually taste the water.

Lunch is a major vacation every day in our lives. Have we ever reflected on this? Or, do we eat at our desk thinking we are getting more done? Do we rush out and bring a sandwich back to continue working? Do we work through lunch because our boss does and he expects it from everyone? If so we are actually getting less done, and it is emotionally and physically unhealthy! Without an appropriate lunch vacation our productivity for the afternoon is much less.

At lunch we need to remove ourselves from our work station and refocus. It is best to go outside if even for a few minutes, walk and get fresh air. On appropriate weather days we might consider eating outside in a park or at a nearby table. If we choose to eat at a restaurant, a light meal hearty in fruits and vegetables is best. Large, heavy meals will bring about lethargy in the afternoon. Alcohol should be avoided at lunch because it inhibits optimum afternoon performance. We have now consciously set the stage for an afternoon of productive work and many mini-vacations to look forward to.

Our evenings are also blessed with numerous mini-vacations. Even if we have to make dinner, take the children to piano lessons and so on, each activity is seen as a mini-vacation separate from each of the other activities. We enjoy each one for its own merit taking in the sights, sounds and smells.

Taking dozens of mini-vacations every day is a habit we need to cultivate. It will take a considerable, conscious effort to change a lifetime of self- neglect. The payoff is enormous! With a little creativity each of us can create many mini-vacations that suit the structure of our daily life. With our change in focus and behaviour, it becomes apparent that each day of our lives is really about numerous, joyous vacations interspersed with work. The reality is we are much more productive and happier than ever before.

*Chapter 22*

# Doing Life

## Catastrophizing

There is probably no other behaviour that escalates and perpetuates anxiety and stress faster. Catastrophizing is reacting to feelings and thoughts regarding a situation in such a way as to create the illusion that things are worse than they actually are. Once started, a mixture of thoughts, feelings, behaviours and anxiety continue an upward spiral where we lose sight of reality. The more we engage in the habit of catastrophizing the more difficult it usually is to stop the behaviour. Unless we do stop, and face each moment as it really is, there is little we can do to create an effective stress management program.

Sometimes, we can see this behaviour in ourselves without feedback from others. If on more than one occasion others have suggested we catastrophize then it is almost a sure thing we do. It is so easy to deny what we are being told, but it is prudent for our own good to pay attention to what others are saying. The message may come in the form of: "you make mountains out of an ant hill, you always think the worse, you are so negative, why is it always me, things can't get any worse, things won't get better," or some variation of these themes.

Our task is see things as they actually are, or reframe our thinking until we are in a space that accurately depicts the situation. We need to slowly, methodically and accurately revisit the events of a situation, be aware of all our thoughts and feelings around that situation, and know we are OK. We need to use the awareness of how we have inappropriately learned to react from our thoughts and feelings instead of being with them, while observing what is happening and what needs done. Catastrophizing is often a behaviour learned over many years, and can be firmly entrenched. If we cannot reasonably change this pattern ourselves, it is advisable to obtain appropriate help. The importance of eliminating catastrophizing cannot be overstated.

## Perception Scale

For most us it takes practice to accurately judge the seriousness of a situation. Said differently, it takes practice to not catastrophize, but also not downplaying the gravity of the situation either. It is clear we can improve this skill with practice. Imagine a scale with numbers from one to ten. It is called the perception scale, or the degree to which we accurately assess a situation. Let's assume number ten is the worst possible scenario, whatever that is for you, death of a loved one for example. Lets say number one represents a very minor irritation, whatever that is for most of us.

Begin practising by assigning a number on the scale that best represents the stress of a particular daily situation. An example might be your in-laws coming for dinner. At the end of the day review your perception (scale number) with the flow of events that occurred, and your thoughts and feelings about the event. With practice in different situations we are better able to accurately see the threat of a situation, if any. We gradually learn that when we assign a number to a situation, it is an accurate assessment. We then know what to expect and what actions to undertake. This exercise takes patience, commitment and time, but the rewards are enormous.

# Pamper Yourself

The news continues to get better. View yourself as the king or queen of the land, rich, famous and everyone adores you. Well, you may not be all those things but you are an important part of everything, and are blessed with whatever circumstances you face, no matter how challenging. Actually, it makes no difference if you are the poorest person in the land or a rich queen.

Pamper yourself! This means something different to each of us. Remember, life is simply each moment, now, not dealing with an hour from now or tomorrow. This does not mean we abdicate planning today for what we require tomorrow.

How do I pamper myself at the most intimate level? That is the question for each of us. After all we are important, we are part of the solution in the world, aren't we? If the honest answer seems no, than we have a lot of work to do. If the answer seems yes, let's proceed. The question is, in what thousands of small ways can each of us pamper ourselves?

Pampering does not mean we need to spend much, or indeed any money on ourselves. On the other hand if pampering yourself is buying a new yacht and airplane then go for it. The goal is to enjoy ourselves, or feel good on the simplest and most intimate level possible. It means giving ourselves treats that we might not ordinarily do. It is first giving ourselves permission to treat ourselves. If we enjoy a particular TV program, pampering may be taking one hour a week out of busy family life and enjoying that one program. We are then happier and feel better about ourselves. Most likely we then function better as a spouse and parent.

Pampering is sitting for five minutes enjoying our cup of coffee instead of drinking it while doing something else. It is buying our favourite flavour of coffee once a week instead of our regular daily flavour. It is buying a monthly magazine on an interesting topic, a magazine we might not have otherwise chosen to buy. Pampering is the anticipation of going to the movies next Friday to see the movie we have wanted to see for the past three months. Pampering has two aspects, the action and the anticipation. We receive pleasure from both. Anticipating one bite of chocolate for three days before it happens brings enormous pleasure. Look for endless ways of pampering yourself.

We are very sensual beings. We receive great pleasure from all our senses. So let's use them on a daily basis. Treat yourself to your favourite flavour of ice cream each week. Slowly, taste every drop of ice cream flow over the tongue and then cascade down your throat. Taste like you have never tasted before. A very small amount of ice cream brings tremendous sensual enjoyment. Use your imagination as to what other foods you can use in enjoying the practice.

Our sense of smell is so enjoyable. Light some of your favourite candles,  sit back in a comfortable position and enjoy. Turn on your favourite music if you wish. Open a bottle of your favourite wine to accompany the situation. Another suggestion is enjoying a bubble bath on a regular basis. A professional massage is extremely therapeutic and sensual. Many people have one on a regular basis.

Much of the joy of pampering oneself is being open to new activities. The exploration of pampering will last the rest of your life. As suggested earlier the most difficult task may be giving ourselves permission to behave like this. We may have feelings of guilt, or just a lifetime of other habits filling our days. Begin by consciously choosing pampering exercises on a regular basis. Soon they will be part of the day you can't miss.

## Don't Take It Personally

The world is fast-paced and dynamic. So many things are happening sometimes to us and sometimes to others. It often appears that we have been chosen, picked out or targeted by someone, a group, nature, God, or whatever. Very seldom is this the case.

If someone tells us we are lousy at our job, our first reaction is to take it personally and be upset. In this example, if we react personally the only conclusion is that we are indeed lousy at our job, and we should thank the person for pointing it out. Our task is to do something about being lousy at our job. On the other hand if the accusation is not true it is impossible to take it personally. We know it is not true. There is nothing to be upset about. A statement made by someone else is more about their beliefs and personality. By taking something personally we are agreeing with it.

Nothing other people do is because of us. It is because of themselves. Everyone lives in their own little world completely different from the world each of us live in. If we take something personally we assume they know everything about our world. Well, they know almost nothing! Even when a situation seems personal, a comment or action from another is about their point of view.

We create vast amounts of unnecessary stress for ourselves by taking things personally. With a little consistent practice we can master one of the most powerful stress-busting tools available.

## You Are Not Important

Shocking? This may be a difficult notion to get past. It seems so contrary to the way most of us were raised and how we live our lives. It is virtually impossible to talk or think our way through this. The more we reflect on all things the clearer it becomes. Only then will we have the opportunity to come closer to our true importance.

## Fairness

There is room to suggest that no other issue invites more

stress in our lives than the idea of fairness. Fairness is a belief of the mind, in other words it does not exist. Most of us have been brought up to believe in fairness and to treat others in a fair way, which is a wonderful way of behaving. Often we interpret events as being unfair, but there is no underlying rule, law or supreme orchestrator who evenly distributes the positive and negative events of the world. They happen!

When something happens our reaction is often from our belief system, instead of reality. We believe in fairness instead of seeing reality. We become stuck in our belief and don't institute the action required to deal with a situation. The more we focus on our idea of fairness the more it becomes a habit. It is essential that we get past ideas of fairness. If we are unable to do so it is suggested we seek appropriate help.

## Hope

Hope is a toxic word. When we use this word we are suggesting we are not facing the facts. It is a way of escaping the pain of feeling and thinking about the possible outcomes. Often it prevents us from taking appropriate action. Hoping suggests a divine intervention will rescue us. It sets us up for more disappointment if we don't receive the desired outcome.

We need to see all the facts and possible outcomes of a situation. Next we focus on what needs to be done. It is helpful to notice when we use the word hope in our thinking and speaking. We might ask ourselves how we can rephrase our comment by including all outcome possibilities and our action taken. Then we are free to discuss our preferred outcomes.

## Multitasking

The more stress we are under, the more tasks we take

on at one time. We rush more and more, and for a while it appears we are doing what needs done. It does not work! We are making more errors, and physically and emotionally wearing ourselves down for future endeavours. Overall efficiency dramatically declines.

The issue is we believe we can do many things at once, and the more we are in the stress cycle, the greater our illusion is reinforced. We need to make deliberate conscious choices. As previously discussed, we need to prioritize and consciously choose one action at a time. This takes practice. One thing at a time is the only sane way to live life.

## Important vs Urgent

This dilemma is caused by a lack of clarity in our lives. It comes from reacting emotionally instead of clearly seeing the facts. On a piece of paper create two columns with the above headings and write in as many scenarios as you can think of in each column. This exercise will give a starting point in discerning what is urgent and important. Of course life isn't the neat list we create in our minds.

Urgent means things need attended to now. Important means things must be attended to soon, they can't be dismissed. With practice we better learn to discern between the two. We need to act on situations with a balance of emotion and reason.

## Is vs Should

Notice how often we use the word *should* in our thinking and speaking. It represents the degree to which we are not facing the facts, and hoping a mystical power creates the mythical situation our mind has created. We cannot do what needs done while focusing on what the ideal situation might be, and spending unnecessary energy. We meet the challenge by clearly seeing the facts. Practice moving from a position of what *should* be, to what *is* and notice how much more effective you are in dealing with situations.

## Believe Nothing Or No One

Live each moment as a clean slate, as if you just arrived here on earth and have so much to learn. Find out for yourself and listen to no one. Learn from moment-to-moment first hand experience. Then you are not ingesting someone else's interpretation of what life is. They don't know, they only have an opinion. The more they claim to know, the more they are lost.

Stated differently, earnestly question everyone and everything. We can't literally go through life not trusting, that's impossible because we are in relationship with all things. The point is, be very sure what is happening based on your own interaction with life. Now you are completely responsible for your subsequent actions, there is no one else to blame. Chances are your actions are now based on a far more realistic view of the world.

## Don't Be A Follower

This comment relates to the one above. Each of us lives the same life under our skin. We all have the same thoughts and feelings. We all feel stress to a greater or lesser degree. We just look and sound different on the outside, which is misleading. To behave the same as someone else is to bring the same result, the same life as they have. Who wants to be like them?

The more we see things for ourselves the more we realize others are lost, and create their own stress. The only natural thing to do is not follow them, but follow our own view of the world and be a trailblazer. Try it! Simple joy and contentment will immediately follow.

## Balance In Decision Making

The following quote is taken from Malcolm Gladwell's book, *blink*: "truly successful decision making relies on a balance between deliberate and instinctive thinking." The second part of the quote from the same author states, "in good decision making, frugality matters." In other words, reduce a complex situation to its simplest elements. Almost everything has an identifiable underlying pattern.

## Gossip

Gossip is the fuel of stress for ourselves and others. In the large view it is destructive for all concerned. It contributes nothing! When confronting gossip, a simple response might be, "I have no need to know this information" and walk away. Do you notice how you are taking more control in life? Notice how others start treating you differently?

## Nature

The woods, meadows, streams and so on are a product of the universe, larger picture, God or however we choose to describe it. Each of us is also the same product, or flow. So often we lose sight of this, and separate ourselves off with individual problems, stress, thinking, an inflated ego, and so on. One of the most powerful stress busters available is to simply return to nature.

Go for a walk in nature and return to your natural home. Use all your senses. Look, smell, physically touch the leaves, listen to the sounds and let go. Notice the relationship among all things. Of course, we are quiet. Notice how difficult this might be? When our thoughts turn to work, worries, and so on gently return to noticing the walk. Make it a practice to return to nature each day. At work it may consist of a walk in the park after lunch, or at home a walk in the evening after dinner. Albert Einstein understood when he said, "look deeply into nature, and then you will understand everything better."

Notice how we are not the same person as before. We are

now better prepared to return to our responsibilities of life.

## Never Give Up

The only time we give up or quit is at the moment of our death. Then it is officially over. Take the instinctive view animals have, they fight until their death. A situation may seem stressful, challenging or even hopeless but remember we only have to deal with this moment. Things change, we make them change! Right now allow it to be part of your core being,  never give up.

This attitude includes constantly reviewing situations and taking different action.

## Failure

When we were unsuccessful at a particular task we often see ourselves as failures. We might safely say we failed at that particular task. The issue rises when we generalize and see ourselves as failures in many areas. We conclude we cannot succeed at anything. That is not a fact. The fact is we failed at one particular task. Look at the successful tasks we have completed. They are the facts.

After each failure we have an opportunity to begin again with a clean slate, and usually with more wisdom. In other words, a failure gives us the opportunity for a fresh start each time in life. It can't get any better than that! Take this view now and carry it with you forever.

## Change

It is natural that change induces stress in most people. A change in jobs, moving homes, retirement and so on need to be seen as situations where stress symptoms might naturally arise. We are changing routines, surroundings, friends and facing unknowns. These are ingredients of stress. Ahead of time take control of the things you can control and look for the wonderful new opportunities that might soon arise. Prepare an arsenal of stress busters you can draw upon when needed. Surprises will surface, but you already know this, so they won't be surprises. Deal with them!

## Nutrition

This may be the most over publicized topic in the media today, making it the most confusing. The facts are simple: appropriate nutritional habits are critical for optimum physical and mental health, which is also critical in stress reduction.

There are countless books, programs, diets and gurus all claiming they have the answer. They don't! The author endorses no diets, books, programs or gurus. Stay away from all these.

Rigourously educate yourself on the nutritional needs of the body. This includes what the body requires and what all foods have to offer. Know your body and its exceptional needs, either from first hand experience or trusted medical advice. Be acutely aware of food intake balancing energy output. Through trial and error and careful planning, tailor a nutritional program to best suit your needs.

This exercise takes tremendous commitment and work. It is a long term project. There are no short cuts. The pay off is enormous.

## Exercise

Humans are animals that have evolved over millions of years in the same way all others have evolved. Animals have evolved to be active; they run, jump, crawl, fly, swim and play. By our very nature we are intended to do these things. The body maintains optimum health when it vigourously works on a regular basis. Doing what is natural is the ultimate stress buster.

The dilemma is similar to nutrition. We have separated ourselves from the issue of what it is to be human and natural. Too many people have too much to say about the topic of exercise. Most don't know! We are bombarded with advice from all corners of the media. There are countless programs on aerobic, anaerobic, weight bearing exercises, yoga, pilates, and more out there. You can even pay a personal trainer but chances are they don't know either.

Know what activities you enjoy. Find out if you don't know. This list may include walking, running, skiing, cycling, skating, hiking, mountain climbing, canoeing, and so on. The list is as long as your imagination. Rigourously educate yourself about exercise biomechanics and physiology. Educate yourself about various ways of obtaining appropriate levels of aerobic and anaerobic exercise. Find out the many ways of practicing weight bearing exercises.

Use numerous daily activities combining your passions with meeting the requirements of the body. Of course these activities are based on a sound understanding of your health and trusted medical advice.

Rigourous regular exercise is considered one of the best antidotes to stress. Make it part of your daily routine just like eating. Learn to play, be an animal, you are one!

## Controllable vs Not Controllable

The sensible person doesn't waste time and energy trying to control feelings, thoughts and events that have already happened. We can't control what happens to someone who had a serious accident. It's over. Let the doctors do their work. Explore what options are available to, or controllable by you now. Choose and move on. It does not mean you don't have feelings about what happened. Acknowledge them and take action.

The skill of discerning and appropriately acting on what is controllable and letting go of what is not controllable is a very major stress buster. It is a skill that you will carry with you for life. It takes practice to fine tune this skill. Notice little daily events that happen and internally practice by asking yourself in which of the two above categories they belong. With practice you will be more prepared to handle the larger events of life.

## Baby Steps

Some days in life are challenging. We don't know how to deal with a situation or don't think anything we do will help. Remember the prisoners of war? This was reality for them. When not sure, move slowly, cautiously because maybe this approach won't work. Maybe we have to change plans or actions, that's OK, that's the essence of life. In other words baby steps may be the answer.

We have so much to learn from the young. A baby is determined and committed to walk. They are as inexperienced in this present moment as we are but it does not matter. Falling and scraping themselves, they move about their task as if it is predetermined that they will succeed. They will, so will we. They take one step at a time, and that's all we need to do in any situation. Taking baby steps will bring about what is best for us in the end. We may have a different opinion about the result, but our opinion is not important. That is the mark of an evolved person.

When we are not sure, take baby steps.

## Role Models

Most of us at some time in our lives have looked at someone and asked, "why can't I be like him/her? They can handle this." There are many remarkable people in life and we have a lot to learn from them. It is appropriate to see others as role models and an opportunity to learn from them. There is also great danger. We must not in any way turn power over to them, idolize them, or emulate them.

Our task is crawl under their skin and see how/why they operate. What world views do they hold? What self-esteem do they carry? What is their attitude in life? What coping skills do they carry with them? What level of self-importance do they carry? How does their sense of resilience and hardiness manifest? The questions are endless. Always be looking for role models, but be careful. Now you are the role model for someone else.

## Normalize

When we are going through challenging, difficult times we often feel alone. We tell ourselves, that we are the only person this is happening to, we can't cope. It seems that way, but it is not true. Sometimes it helps to share with or listen to people in similar circumstances. It may be once or twice, or long term. We quickly realize that we are not alone, this challenge is part of life and many people are facing it. We normalize the situation instead of viewing it as an aberrant attack on ourselves.

Seek out friends who have had similar experiences. If none are available spread out your search by asking your doctor, community mental health services, support groups, and so on. If there are no support groups for what you are looking for in your community start one yourself. What a wonderful example of empowering yourself and taking control. Look at all the others you are helping too.

## Needs vs Wants

This often unrecognized dilemma is a major source of stress in our lives. What we need in life are the basics - food, water, clothing, air, and shelter. We have lost sight of this and gravitate to what pleases us on a superficial level. We mistakenly include these things in our needs list. These are simply our wants. We continue to strive for wants instead of settling for needs. Tremendous conflict, turmoil and stress results.

The prisoners of war were quickly forced to face this issue. They were stripped emotionally and physically and realized what was needed, which they rarely had. They pined for the very basics of life, and were so content if they thought for a moment they would come close to having the basics. They couldn't imagine having or wanting any more.

Our task is to return, to a more basic way of living, always being aware of what we need and what we want. The awareness alone reduces stress significantly because we consciously decide if our choice emanates from a need or want. There is no stress around the resulting choice. There is nothing wrong with obtaining wants (being very rich for example) as long as we are clear it is a want, and we are responsible for the results.

In small ways practice listing things that you acquire as needs or wants. You may start with gum, cup of coffee, new socks and so on. It may seem trivial at first but continue to work on as many items as possible. Over time you will have greater clarity around this issue and be better prepared to make decisions.

## Celebrate The Miracles Of Today

No matter what the challenge of the moment, it is within a greater context. Step outside your personal view, even for a moment if possible. The universe is constantly changing, galaxies are exploding and evolving, stars are dissolving, trees are blossoming, insects are buzzing, babies are born, people are dying, snow is falling, and we are still here in flesh. Wonderful! We are the continuous evolution of the universe, from the distant galaxies, to the birth of the baby robin, to our own breathing, we are simply part of it. Wow, we are here! Life is a miracle! Each moment is a miracle!

When we choose to be present with this, the pettiness of our lives returns to its proper place. When under stress, sit back, take a deep breath, practice stress reduction techniques, and celebrate the miracles of today. Albert Einstein said it better than most of us, "There are only two ways to live your life. One is as though nothing is a miracle. The other is as though everything is a miracle."

## Pretend

Regularly we are in stressful challenging situations. Life is like that. Sometimes it is helpful to pretend our desired outcome has already happened, in other words fake it. There is an immediate shift in our attitude and perception. We seem able to better cope. Chances are, things that need to happen will happen now.

If your boss seems impossible, doesn't listen, doesn't care, is rude, demanding, self-centred, just pretend it often works. Pretend your your boss is everything you wish for in a boss, empathetic, supportive, listens, is proactive and so on. Treat and talk with him/her in this context. Watch for extraordinary results.

## Transpose Positions

Sometimes when in difficult challenging situations it is helpful to transpose our position. We then momentarily change our view. Often this is enough to create space in the larger picture to see things differently.

Suppose you have an ongoing difference of opinion with your mother. It is a chronic irritating situation. Transpose your position for a moment and ask how I would see this if I were in her position? What a revelation! Now do what needs done.

## Confidence

Mary has the confidence to handle this, I don't. This is too difficult. I can't do it, I don't have the confidence. We live with mistaken identity. We assume confidence is inbred, a natural gift we have from the beginning. The reality is confidence comes from succeeding, no matter what the cost. Then we know we can succeed in the future.

If you don't have confidence, get some by doing what needs done this moment, no matter what the cost. Earn it, it's not free.

## Apologize

It is best to do things appropriately the first time. Unfortunately, sometimes we don't and create problems. Apologize when needed. It is so easy to avoid or pretend we did not do something. Well, the rest of the world knows anyway! Apologizing says to everyone that we are sensitive and aware of our impact on the world. Obviously to be of any worth in life we need this quality. Apologizing suggests our ego is intact, in other words it is a way of normalizing ourselves and admitting we are no better than others.

Apologizing says I have learned from this mistake and it will never happen again. We build integrity. People see our growth and continue to change  how they treat us.

## Make A difference

Each of us is an integral part of life. We are here right now, so we are important. It is too easy to say I can't do anything, I am not a politician, a doctor, or whatever. We have all made this statement, with our own personal view of what we can't do.

Make a difference right now by picking up a piece of litter from the road. Notice the thoughts and feelings. Reflect on the impact towards others of this simple act. We have thousands of opportunities each day to make a difference. While walking we can smile to a stranger, hold the door for someone, or thank someone from the heart. How can we experience stress while behaving like this? We have turned attention away from ourselves and have extended it outwards.

Seek volunteer positions in your community. Spending only several hours a week volunteering will create a refreshing, rejuvenating view of life. William James told us, "Act as if what you do makes a difference. It does."

## Media

It is so simple to view life through coloured glasses. What is reality? We saw it on TV, read it, saw it on the internet, heard it, or simply believe it. Who knows? Marshall McLuhan was credited with saying, "the medium is the message." In other words, how do we create the reality of our world? He is suggesting our world is simply the medium through which we were delivered ideas. So is our reality simply what we are bombarded with through the media? Then what do we really know? What is really going on?

At no other time in the evolution of mankind have we been more bombarded with "media news." We ingest what we are bombarded with, then interpret it to suit our individual needs. We are confused. So what is reality? Imagine living one, two or three hundred years ago. How did we learn what was going on? How fast did the information arrive? Did it arrive? How much did we care? Did we live in our community or some fictional far off place? Did we know about our immediate community, who lived in it? How did we know? This last question is critical. Were we overwhelmed by media bombardment, or did we have to rely on direct experience? Then how did we interpret events?

One of our great sources of stress today is addiction to media. Information is coming so quickly our nervous systems cannot handle it. Our cognitive processes cannot deal with it. Accuracy of everything is questionable. We have become information junkies. At best, everything is someone else's interpretation. It is about what someone else wants us to think. What role does direct experience have?

We need to slow down, step back, turn off the TV, turn off the computer, turn off the cell phone, put the newspaper down, stop listening to others and begin to live life. What is that? You are about to find out! There is no greater stress buster.

## Pay The Price

The world is constantly changing, so our lives are different each moment. There are more demands than ever being thrust upon us, at work, home and from society in general. Each moment we must re-negotiate our lives due to changing circumstances. Remember the elastic band? It can only expand so far. Often we are stretching ourselves too thin. We have  responsibility to do something before it is too late.

When we have done everything possible, then it is time to pay the price. That means walk away, quit the job, move to another geographical location, or whatever it takes. There will be a significant loss or price to pay. It may be a financial loss, personal loss, loss of title at work, loss of self-image, loss of professional status, or loss of friends. It will be painful but worth it. Sometimes we must take a step back in order to continue moving forward.

When we choose to continue in a downward spiral with stress, we are saying we are not worthy of a better life, we are only meant to struggle. Really? We are saying we are so important the world can't survive without us. Really? The athlete doesn't experience success without paying a price. We don't raise a family without paying a price. We don't pass an exam without paying a price. Someone has arrived at a certain level of development when they are present with the notion that no price is too high to pay for an appropriate life.

## All vs Nothing

Some of us have polarized ourselves in many ways. This

shows up in behaviour such as we must be the the best at everything, or not try. We must be the top person or not be involved. We must look the smartest, be the prettiest, and so on or not be there. The more we have polarized ourselves, or live from extreme positions, the more stress we create for ourselves.

We spend great energy trying to be at one end of a self-created scale. We create internal conflict and tension attempting to reconcile the dissonance between who we are and who we think we should be. This means stress. Most of us are average in most things. It is important for each of us to face this reality, and inquire as to why we set unrealistic standards.

## Communication

Misunderstanding what someone said, or withholding something that needs said are powerful stressors. In other words our communication needs to be clear, precise and to the point. We can be left with no doubts about what was said in a conversation. Sometimes this is not easy. We draw conclusions, then act on what we believe was said or meant or what we wanted to hear. This creates confusion and conflict.

It is highly recommended the reader sensitize themselves to what is needed to improve their communication skills. In any conversation be willing to ask the speaker to clarify what they meant. Reframe or paraphrase something someone said in order to see if that is what they actually meant.

## Passive vs Assertive

Often there is a fine line between doing too little in a situation and doing what is required. Doing what is required, absolutely no more or no less is being assertive. This is a stress buster. Doing less than what is needed is being passive, and creating stress. With practice in a variety of situations we learn to ascertain what is assertive behaviour.

We are deemed aggressive in a situation when doing more than what is required. This is unnecessary and unhealthy for all concerned.

## Everything To All

The sense, we must be loved by everyone and everyone must approve of everything we do, is a major stressor. This position is stupid and irrational because it is impossible! Rather we should seek other people who more closely share values and interests with us. A powerful way of being in life is to maintain our own personal integrity, being true to our own values, while striving to be loving, creative, productive and contributing individuals.

When we do that we let people like us or not as they choose, and not be overly anxious about it.

## Avoidance

It is easier to avoid difficulties and responsibilities in life than to face them. By doing so we create more and worse problems in the future. It is best to face problems squarely and solve them to the best of our ability. Putting things off only increases our anxiety and depression. We build confidence and happiness by living life here and now. Remember, what needs to be done now?

## Take Risks

We need to live life as openly as possible. This helps us avoid repeating the same things over and over, and living in the same dimension. Don't always play it safe. We open ourselves to new experiences and possibilities when we take risks. We move to other realms. Life is an adventure.

We create undue stress will attempting to overly protect

ourselves. Of course wisdom prevails, seat belts and bicycle helmets are probably  good things.

## Thought Stopping

Sometimes we are simmering inside about an issue. The voices in our head are speaking at an ever increasing pace. There becomes a point when we literally have to intervene with ourselves in order to bring this to a halt. We might talk to ourselves out loud or sub vocally. Nevertheless we say STOP this now. We might visualize a STOP sign while doing so. We keeping repeating this until the the voices stop carrying on.

## Be Creative

When we are in touch with the vastness of our core existence as human beings, there are no boundaries or limits. We are stripped of our need to focus on ourselves and things that we think are wrong. Be creative! Try it, it works. Sing a song, make up a poem, pick up a paint brush, make something different for dinner, start knitting, buy a different brand of wine, learn a new dance, do woodworking, the list will only end when you die.

There is no beginning or end when we create. There is only constantly creating, being new and open to the moment, having fun. There is no person who is constantly creating that has many perceived dilemmas with associated stress. Make a commitment to spend some time each day being creative. Don't know what to do? Pick something you enjoyed or were passionate about as a child. It's always a great starting point.

## Worst Case Scenario

In difficult situations sometimes it is helpful to look at the worse case scenario. What is the worst outcome that can happen here? We squarely face this in our mind. We know we can handle it. If you think you can't, of course you can, you have learned this by now. We find a way to handle anything, by our resilience, with our basket of coping tools and meeting the needs of the moment.

Chances are, of course, the worst case scenario will not happen and an outcome of much lesser consequence will happen. So you are prepared because you were prepared for the worst. It is getting easier and easier to cope.

## Say No

When we mean no, say **No.**

## Many Solutions

Often we think there is one perfect solution to every dilemma. If it is not found we assume a disaster is looming. This is irrational thinking because there are many possible solutions to most dilemmas, and rarely is there a perfect one. Each solution has its strengths and weaknesses. The best we can do is pick one of the better ones and give it a try. If it does not work we pick another one. We live by doing the best we can in any given circumstance. Over time things generally go well. If we hold out for the perfect solution decisions are made by default, and generally these are not the best.

## Be Open to Boredom

Most of us fear boredom. We live perpetually busy lives continually on automatic. We don't dare slow down and look at ourselves. Why? Each of us knows the thoughts and feelings that will arise. At all costs we avoid facing them. So we keep busy. There is continuous friction between keeping a lid on not looking at our life, and maintaining busyness. The result is chronic stress, which often we are not even aware of.

Those times we have nothing to do, maybe even wanting something to do is a wonderful opportunity. On the surface boredom seems unnatural, we have feelings and thoughts about doing this and that, we should be busy, and so on. Be open to boredom! Be with the uncomfortable feelings of boredom. Be with the thoughts and feelings that arise. Use them to face the life that is avoided. Soon boredom won't seem uncomfortable, but will be a friend. Observe wonderful changes in your life.

## Get a Pet

Pets are the masters at giving unconditional love, and being open to receiving endless amounts of love. Appropriately caring for a pet is a major stress buster. While our focus is turned towards loving and caring for a pet on a daily basis we cannot be focused on ourselves. Walking, playing with, and cuddling with a pet is soothing and relaxing. The bond of affection is second to none. Your pet will endlessly listen to you talk about your life, and never judge or talk back.

Getting a pet must be seen as a major commitment. Your pet requires significant amounts of daily play and care. It requires ongoing medical care. If one is not committed to meet the demands of being a pet owner then the decision should be made to not proceed.

## Negativity

One of the most toxic poisons to a healthy quality of life is negative people. We recognize them the moment we are near them. They have nothing good to say about anyone (except themselves) or the world. They play helpless and are master manipulators in getting others to join their cause of being helpless and blaming. Unfortunately this behaviour spreads like a fire. Others are quick to join.

Each of us creates the world with our behaviour, so with negative people around the quality of our circumstances is deteriorating quickly. We have a responsibility to put a stop to this behaviour. As always, we are modelling a completely different behaviour. Sometimes this may have an effect on them. We have a responsibility to speak with them and invite them to more closely look at their attitude and behaviour. If all fails, get away from them. Leave! Otherwise we will be very quickly pulled to their level, which is what they want. We have much to offer the world and we must be committed to move on without negativity. This attitude is a major stress buster.

## Rescuing

Rescuing involves trying to change people who are not taking the interest, or making the effort to change themselves. Even if someone really should stop smoking or spend more time with their family you can't force them to change. Rescuing is about having inappropriate boundaries on our part. It is about not looking at what changes we need to make in ourselves. It is about imposing our will on someone else. It is about swimming against the tide when inappropriate.

By its very nature this behaviour produces chronic frustration and conflict. We are never going to be successful. It is a major stressor for ourselves, and our chronic stress continually impacts on those around us. Sometimes rescuing is subtle, and difficult to notice in ourselves. It is masked by thoughts of "doing the right thing" or "just helping." This issue often resolves around not wanting to look at our own thoughts, feelings, low self-esteem, or inflated ego. Very often rescuing is associated with the need to be rescued ourselves, which is a major stressor by itself. Feedback from others sometimes helps us see this behaviour. When resolved, a major weight is lifted off our shoulders and the shoulders of those around us.

# Chapter 23
## *Moving On*

We have become very habitual in our thinking and actions. We copy those around us. We listen to the words of our language and immediately create images in our mind of what they mean. We divide our life into categories or divisions and then supply different weights and importance to each division. For example we use the word *career* to describe our job, *family* to describe immediate relatives, *friends* to describe a particular group of people, *hobbies* as something we do when not busy, and so on. We have arbitrarily ranked, or ordered these in importance in our mind. We create vast conflict and stress in daily life trying to maintain the status of these subjectively ordered words and images.

What would happen if we did not have these divisions in our lives? In other words there were no more divisions, or pigeon holes called career, that was separate from family, hobbies, and so on? How could we then put such enormous importance on one thing such as our career (and accompanying stress), and forgo hobbies and family? For some strange reason we have decided to live our lives in parts, each with different meaning.

What would happen if we saw our life as one continuous flow, or movement? There being no divided parts, every action being related to every other action, nothing having undue importance, living with the flow of the moment. Put differently, we have separated ourselves off from life by creating all our divisions and seeing no connection between events. Sometimes for the sake of communication it is prudent to use dividing words such as career. But the key is to be aware the words are only used temporarily for conversation.

We arrive on earth in flesh, and will soon leave the earth. Everything is movement. The galaxies and stars are constantly being born and dying. The trees, flowers, animals and so on are replacing the ones before them. Everything that exists is changing and moving. We **are** this change, movement, or flow. What would life be like for us if we were in touch with this? Why not begin a rigourous inquiry now? William James told us, "human beings can alter their lives by altering their attitudes of mind."

Because everything is changing, we undergo an evolutionary rejuvenation as we become more adept at dealing with stress. We become different people by learning better coping techniques, seeing the world differently, having a different relationship with everything, and building confidence that we can handle life. In other words, success breeds success. Our confidence level grows exponentially. We literally change as a human being, from the the inside out.

As we dramatically change we have an impact on those around us. We are empowered by being with the natural flow of all things. We are not internally divided by thinking and giving words so much meaning. We don't expect life to be this way or that way. Instead we have more simple fun, do what needs done, and we are more responsible than ever to live an appropriate life which contributes to a better world. Those around us now treat us in a different manner. We create life, we are life!

I am always with myself, and it is I who am my tormentor.
Leo Tolstoy

When we complain about stress, and aren't doing
anything about it, the stress isn't severe enough.
The Author